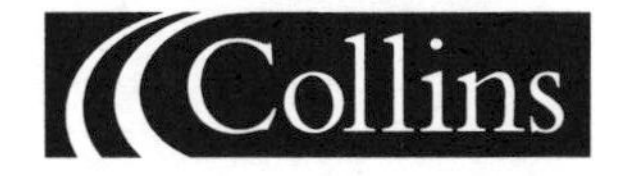

Julia Carling
Kate Shapland

Beauty Scoop.

The indisponsable guide to the best beauty products on the market

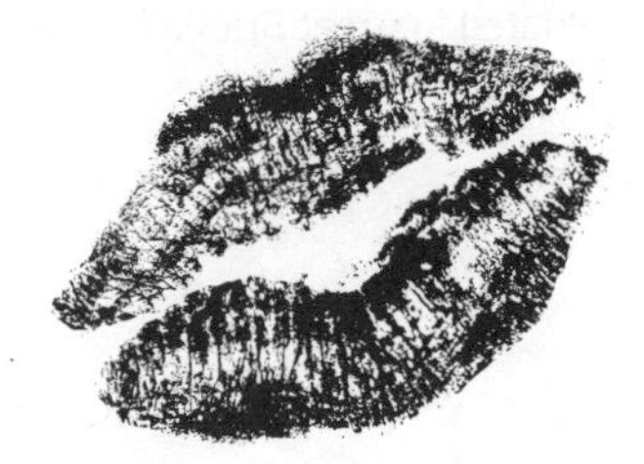

First published in 2004 by
HarperCollins*Publishers*
77-85 Fulham Palace Road
Hammersmith
London W6 8JB

The Collins website address is www.collins.co.uk

09 08 07 06 05 04 03
7 6 5 4 3 2 1

Editor: Joanna Carreras
Designer: Bob Vickers

A catalogue record for this book is available from the British Library

ISBN 0-00-717393-8

Printed in Great Britain by Clowes Ltd, London and Beccles

CONTENTS

INTRODUCTION: welcome to a mumbo-jumbo free zone

First, a question: how often have you wondered whether the £20 or £30 you have just splashed out on a new face cream or foundation could have been better spent?

By that we don't mean do you think you could have got more mileage out of £30-worth of groceries (we are talking here about spending money on *yourself*); we mean, does it ever cross your mind that the money could have been more wisely spent on another moisturiser or foundation – one that would do even more favours for your skin?

We are certain that this is something 99 per cent of you have wondered in the past – otherwise, let's face it, you would not have bought our book. In fact we would go so far to say that we don't believe any woman ever buys beauty products with the complete confidence (let alone conviction) that she has invested in the right ones.

We know this because as beauty writers and broadcasters, the big question everyone relentlessly asks us – no matter what their age, social or cultural background – is 'what is the best anti-ageing moisturiser/anti-cellulite cream/self-tanner?'.

We also have the facts right in front of us. If proof were ever needed that a beauty book which tells it like it is is long overdue, we got it from the 257 people who completed our beauty survey and tried products for us.

Quite simply, we wrote this book because you asked us to. There is a genuine and pressing need for straightforward, objective advice on beauty. To say this is hard to come by is an understatement. *It barely exists!* And as the market gets bigger – with more 'solutions' for more 'problems' – and the more mega bucks are at stake, the less likely it is that you will ever get impartial advice on beauty products. Which is hardly fair. Why should you be expected to spend your hard-earned cash on products on which you can only ever get a one-sided view? Music, film, books and even fashion have their critics. Car buyers have Jeremy Clarkson for goodness sake!

So what happens with beauty? You find yourself standing in a chemist's aisle or a busy perfumery department, trying to remember the name of the mascara you read about in a magazine last month so you can go to the counter and buy it without having to ask for advice. You know that if you do you will be interrogated about your beauty routine, given some flannel about the scientific side of products (this is *you* speaking, not us!) and leave with two or three products you don't need.

The women who did our survey wrote honestly about their beauty shopping experiences because we asked them to. And we got back comments like: 'I ignore beauty counter advice because I know it's biased', 'I've been ripped off so often by expensive products that have been misleading with their claims', 'I'm not interested in paying for advertising and marketing', and 'the pressure and heavy sales talk at counters is off-putting'. At the same time though, many of the same people admitted that they are 'never sure' what their skin type is, they *love* luxurious packaging, and that although they know good skin/hair/body shape mainly comes comes down to genes, they still want miracle products that 'get rid of' wrinkles and cellulite.

These remarks – the tip of iceberg – were typical, and spoke volumes to us about the *status quo* of the market, your understanding of it and of beauty generally.

So our challenge was to separate the fluff from the fact and tell you all that we have picked up (at least as much as we could cram into one book) about beauty – what works and what doesn't – to help you become an informed beauty consumer.

As well as this, we wanted to tell you which products are really worth your money and we decided the best way to find this out was to ask *you* to test them for us.

The results people got from products would always be subjective: what works for one person may not work so well for another. But interestingly we found that on the whole, the same – if not very similar – positive verdicts came back for the same products. And if a product got full marks (ten out of ten) from at least three testers who felt it met our criteria – as a direct result of road testing it for us or having used it previously – we felt that this was enough to warrant a place in the book.

We stuck religiously to this rationale on road-tested products, making the lives of our publisher and the book's designer hell by refusing to compromise – or follow the conventional format of 'top five' or 'top ten' – simply to ease page layout design.

We went to great lengths to ensure that the information in this book is as accurate as possible but because the business is so fickle and changeable we can't guarantee that all the products mentioned will still be the same price – or exist at all – after publication. If this is the case we can only apologise now and hope that you will find another gem (or two) in the book that makes up for the frustration.

So what was in it for us?

Our motives have always been the same: we realise that you are increasingly overwhelmed by the choices that face you so we wanted to give you the edge on an ever more complex business and empower you as a beauty consumer. Also, as the business has changed and become more controlled by money, so have our roles as beauty journalists, so it has been liberating to write a beauty book that tells it like it is.

What you find on the following pages is 100 per cent genuine.

our road-test rationale

1. **why did we ask non-experts to test the products?** We felt that the people who were going to buy the products should be the people who tested them as anyone directly involved in the beauty business may not be able to assure a 100 per cent impartial verdict. This was The People's Road Test, and although we nearly lost count several times, a total of 257 testers helped us achieve this goal. We also included some of the products we are currently using (which, as it happens, some of our testers rated highest too) because we felt this would give a broad and balanced view of the best – as tested by experts and non-experts.
2. **how many products did we test?** When we asked the people who did our survey whether a book like this would be useful to them, most (but not all!) said yes, but several said only if we were going to review *every single product on the market*. Um .. We managed approximately 2,000 products – covering all categories, except tools of the trade; this we compiled ourselves by drawing on the experience we have gained from working with beauty professionals. The reason for this was either that there was not

sufficient competition for a product, or one product (be it a nail buffer or tweezers) stood out as being clearly superior, or it was not practical to test the products (there was little point, for example, in sending out 50 hairdryers when we already knew which one best met the criteria for a top dryer).

This is how the number of assessed products broke down for each section:

- **body care**: over 200 products – including 64 body moisturisers, 27 body exfoliators and 36 anti-cellulite/body-contouring treatments.
- **skin care**: over 300 products – 25 cleansers and 154 face creams – including active anti-ageing ones and standard day and night lubricants.
- **make-up**: over 600 cosmetics, including 95 foundations, 121 nail polishes and 63 mascaras.
- **hair care**: over 300 products, including 85 shampoos and 160 styling gels waxes, sprays, creams, serums and pomades.
- **nail care** – over 100 products, including 16 nail-strengthening treatments.
- **sun care** – over 200 products in total, including 36 self-tanners alone.

3. **what was the test criteria?** This varied for each product group and we have clarified the criteria within each road-test section. As a rule of thumb though we asked our testers to vote for products that did what they said they would and were effective; were a pleasure to use, and – because many of our testers said it matters so much – a pleasure to look at too.
4. **how did people give us their verdicts?** We prepared questionnaires for everyone who was testing products to complete. And as well as writing (and phoning to tell us) in as much detail as possible what they thought of the products they tried, we asked them to tell us about themselves – what brands they liked, their beauty shopping habits and experiences, what their dream products were, and so on. Verdicts were posted back to us from all over the world: we had guinea pigs in France, Spain, Hong Kong, America and even Australia, and Julia had boxes and boxes of completed questionnaires in her house, some of which (we have to admit) made us roar with laughter.
5. **why didn't we tell you about the really bad products?** A couple of people asked us if we would include in the book products that performed so badly they were not worth buying. But we felt this would waste valuable space that could otherwise be filled with expert advice or good product recommendations, and took the decision only to include positive information.

SKIN CARE

Of all the things that are said about beauty (quite a lot of which are complete baloney), the truest is that your skin care routine should be as simple as you can make it.

So why is it made out to be so complicated?

Because your face has the lion's share of 'problems', that's why. Think about it: as well as spots and dry patches, there are wrinkles and fine lines, patchy pigmentation, sagging, crepyness, 'big' pores and the 'problem' skin types – oily and dry – to deal with. And if we are to believe all we read, every one of these is treatable with cosmetics. Added to this there is a lot of money to be made if a beauty company can make us believe that their products will make us more beautiful and not age so fast.

'if your wrinkles aren't the knock-on effect of too much sun, you can blame your parents: genes are the main influence on the way your skin looks, changes and ages'

No wonder so many of you are confused about what you can expect and achieve with skin care products. The responses we got to our survey show that you are not very clear about basic stuff such as your skin type (are you oily, dry or combination – or all three at different times of the month or year?), how long you should use a product before you see a positive difference in your skin (one reason why lots of you like products which give instant results – because you can actually *see something happening*), and in which order you should be tackling problems like dark circles, puffiness, wrinkles and sagging.

What you need is some long overdue objective advice – which is exactly what we are here to give – as well as impartial opinions on the products that work best – which is what our testers (women like yourselves) have supplied. This is the only way to cut through the hype and find out how to give your skin what it needs without wasting money on products that will just gather dust in your bathroom.

If you want the most unbiased advice on skin care and products, this book will provide it.

What you will find out about in this chapter:

- That products which claim to minimise your pores are a complete con
- Why you have still got dark under-eye circles despite using eye cream
- Which moisturisers are best for your skin *right now*
- Whether anti-ageing treatments get rid of wrinkles (you asked!)
- Whether expensive creams are best (and how much money goes on packaging)
- Which cleansers to avoid like the plague
- How a humble flannel can help your skin look younger
- Why you think you are addicted to lip balm

cleansers

To say that good cleansing is important to your skin is an understatement. Skin which is properly and regularly cleansed looks 100 percent better than skin which gets treated to the odd lather-up every so often with the household soap or swiped with a cleansing wipe – the kind of cleanser many of our product testers admitted they use to wash their faces.

But although clean skin is a good thing, the *way* you cleanse – the physical act of it – could be said to be even more important and beneficial to your skin. So what is the proper way to cleanse? We will reveal all in this chapter (be prepared for a few surprises), also whether it matters if you use a cleansing cream, gel, emulsion or soap – or a cleanser which 'matches' your skin type or your age.

'don't believe anyone who says your cleanser must be the same brand as your moisturiser'

why good cleansing gives you good skin

Cleansing keeps skin clean, yes. But if you do it properly (and twice a day whether or not you have been wearing make-up) this isn't the only benefit:

- cleansing gets your circulation going, bringing fresh blood to the surface of your skin which makes it pink and plump (read: younger) and feel warm to touch.
- cleansing makes your skin more supple and pliable.
- cleansing prepares your skin for moisturiser because the above benefits all help creams absorb better.

how to cleanse your skin

To get the maximum benefits out of cleansing you have to spend more than a minute doing it – and ideally twice a day. This is how to do it properly:

1. Splash your face with water if you are using a wash-off cleanser. Agitate the cleanser in the palms of your hands.
2. Smooth it over your face and use your fingertips to massage it gently into your skin using small, circular movements all over your face. Using a thumb and finger to gently 'pinch' skin – a method called *le Pince de Jacquet* because it was originally promoted by a French therapist – further enhances circulation.
3. If it is water-soluble, use a face flannel to wipe off cleanser, gently rubbing it in circular movements all over your face to stimulate your skin and soften it.
4. Splash or wipe off residue cleanser, pat skin dry and apply moisturiser straight after to seal in the warmth and pinkness. If rinsing with water, use warm – not too hot or icy cold as these temperature extremes can give delicate skin broken veins.

which cleanser for which skin?

We tend to make a decision about which cleanser is best for our skin based on its consistency – gels are often favoured because they are perceived as being 'fresher' and better for oily skins, and creams are thought to be a creamier, more sympathetic options for dry skins. It's worth remembering though that your skin type can change far more frequently than with the seasons. In fact, if you watch it closely (on a day-to-day basis) you will see that your skin can be oily one day and dry the next. In winter though, more people generally suffer from dry skin because lower temperatures and central heating dehydrate it; in summer, the heat tends to make it oilier. It can also feel dry when you are hungover or tired. So in an ideal world you need a cleanser that suits all skin types – or two different ones to swap around with your skin's moods.

- **water-soluble cleansers** can come as soaps, gels, emulsions, foams and creams and are designed to be washed off with water, so they're ideal if you like to have a bit of a splash-about. They tend to be best-suited to oily or combination skin because water can aggravate very dry and sensitive skin.

- **wipe-off cleansers** can come as cold creams, milks and emulsions and tend to be richer than wash-off ones, which is why (along with the fact that they don't involve using water) many people choose them to clean dry skin.
- **cleansing wipes** – developed to do the whole thing in a jiffy – are impregnated with cleansing ingredients and convenient when you are too tired to face doing the full routine. But you don't get the same skin-enhancing benefits as you do with regular cleansing cream or gel – it's a bit like the difference between polishing leather shoes with sponge-on fluid or boot polish and a cloth.

what makes a great cleanser?

- if it is water-soluble, washes off make-up without leaving your face dry and tight (as some soaps do), or greasy (like some cold creams) with water.
- fragrance-free (but we admit these are hard to find).
- doesn't contain abrasive exfoliating grains: your skin doesn't deserve this kind of boot-camp punishment – being 'scrubbed' every time it's washed – and personally we would not use a cleanser with beta or alpha hydroxy acids (BHAs and AHAs) in it either. Your cleanser should be as gentle, mild and non-abrasive as possible.
- doesn't claim to do anything other than *clean your skin*. Some cleansers try to differentiate themselves from others by saying they have moisturisers in them – suggesting that they won't dry out your skin and even that you don't have to use moisturiser afterwards. But no cleanser should dry out your skin anyway; so if the ingredients that do dry out skin were not in a cleanser in the first place there would be no need to put more emollients into it. Don't get sucked into this marketing talk (unless one of these cleansers genuinely does suit you): cleanser can't nourish your skin *and* clean it. This is as illogical as saying shampoos can clean and condition – neither are on your skin (or hair) for long enough anyway, so the benefits get washed down the plughole.

what's in your cleanser?

Any one of these basic purifying ingredients:

- **coconut** – a natural cleansing agent
- **oatmeal** – soothing and good at absorbing oil
- **detergent** – chemicals such as sodium laureth sulphate
- **olive oil** – used as an alternative to animal fat

do you need toner?

We're not big toner fans, and alcohol-based ones definitely get the thumbs down – they are far too fierce for your skin. Toners first appeared back in the 1970s as alcohol-based 'exfoliators'. They were the world's first skin-smoothers: their alcohol literally burned off the top layer of skin. But now that we have proper face exfoliators we can't see the point of toners because they don't have a role. You don't need toner to shift cleanser and freshen your face because water does that. And toner can't 'close' pores either – no topical product can: pores are not elastic, they are either small or large (and often get that way with age because as your complexion gets thinner the skin around your pores gets thicker and more pronounced – which is why they look bigger and more open). As far as we're concerned the best place for a toner that claims to have an astringent effect on your skin and give your pores a 'workout' is in the bin. Alcoholic or not toner is a waste of money, unless you happen to particularly like the smell of rosewater (which is not that easy to find these days).

'if you prefer toner to water, remember that the word astringent usually means it's alcohol-based and highly likely to be too harsh for your skin'

shopping for cleansers

Before you head for the shops or flash your cash:

1. Decide which cleanser is right for your skin. Generally speaking richer creams are better for dry skins and wash-off gels for oily, but it doesn't always come down to skin type – your life style is a big consideration too.
2. Check out the scent – the product is going on your face, and there is nothing worse than splashing out on a cleanser and finding you don't want to use it because you can't bear the way it smells.
3. Decide whether you are happy with the cleanser's claims: if the one you like claims (breath in) to close pores, moisturise, freshen, smooth *and* tone your skin – find another: no cleanser can do all this satisfactorily.
4. Decide how much you want to spend: most of the cleansers that came out well in our road tests were mid-range, but the cheapies came out well too. This will please two of our testers, Genevieve (35) who said 'big brand cleansers are too expensive and not worth the money', and Deborah (65) who wisely pointed out that 'cheaper cleansers are as good – you just have to use them properly'.

... cleansers we rate:

Julia Spiezia Cleansing Cream (£25.80 for 120ml) and Organic Pharmacy Carrot Butter Cleanser (£15.95 for 65ml): 'I prefer cleansing balms – as I like to wash my face rather than cleanse and tone – and preferably organic ones. These two are brilliant.'

Kate 'Nothing specific. I think the flannel is more important than the brand of cleanser you use, but I tend to go for simple water-soluble creams because you can massage them into your skin properly and wipe them off with a flannel. To me this is the epitome of good cleansing because it gets your circulation going, which makes your skin look pink, plump and young.'

the 7 best face cleansers

the mission To find you the most effective and user-friendly face cleansers on the market.

the criteria Our testers judged the skin cleansers they tried on their ability to improve skin clarity, softness, suppleness (any cleanser that made skin dry and tight got the thumbs down immediately) and radiance. They also judged cleansers on their smell because the people who took part in our survey told us that if a product doesn't smell good it goes in the bin – no matter how good it is.

Eve Lom Cleansing Cream £39.50 for 95ml

The one that beauty editors and celebrities swear by: once tried, they say, the results are never forgotton. And they are right, it is brilliant and it makes you cleanse your face properly. But if you have not got time to do the full routine there is no point buying it. A few of our testers said they didn't think it was worth the money, but the number of people who loved it far outweighed them. 'It's worth every penny,' wrote Sophie (28), 'my skin looks ten times better.' 'It's the logical way to cleanse,' wrote Jackie (34), 'and if you do it properly it works. I don't see how you can go back to ordinary cleansers after using it. It makes cleansing a pleasurable experience.'

the science bit: Not so much a cream as thick balm which you massage into your skin to aid lymphatic drainage (which reduces puffiness) and deeply cleanse skin, and remove with a hot muslin cloth.

Nivea Visage Soft Facial Cleansing Wipes

£4.49 for 25 wipes (available in Refreshing and Gentle varieties)

We don't recommend using wipes every time you cleanse because they only remove surface grime. (And *definitely not* baby wipes – a tip we have often read and Julia admits she uses them: your skin deserves more grown-up treatment than this.) But when you are too knackered to cleanse properly at night – or you are travelling – we cannot deny that wipes are a godsend. This brand proved to be the most gentle (a lot of the wipes we tested stung when used near the eyes) and most effective: 'They're so easy, and one wipe does the job – you don't have to use a couple more,' said Helena (15), 'I think they're magic.' Susie (31) has bought another pack since she tested them and said, 'They're good value for money, nicely scented and soft on my skin.'

the science bit: The wipes contain soothing camomile and micro-sponges which suck up and absorb dirt quickly.

Olay Daily Facials Cleansing Cloths

£5.49 for 30 cloths

Another cleansing brainwave and a convenient way to cleanse, but with the added oomph of water, foam and a slightly-exfoliative weaved cloth. 'You can't beat these for ease – they are the perfect alternative to soap and water,' said Louise (19). 'I keep them by the bath and then just throw the cloth away, no messing about.' Sue (51) has been converted too – 'You can still massage your skin,' she wrote 'and they make your skin feel so clean.' But she added that she wishes 'the plastic container they come in could be squishier so it's easier to pack in a spongebag'.

the science bit: The cloths foam up when you wet them to give skin a soapy wash. They are impregnated with skin buffing beta hydroxy acid (BHA), vitamin E and soothing aloe vera and camomile extracts.

Estée Lauder Rich Results Hydrating Cleanser

£14 for 150ml

Definitely the best cleanser we tested for dry skins. 'It feels like some serious care and attention has gone into making this cleanser,' said Lily (41), 'using it just feels so natural – it's like a second skin. It cleans really well but doesn't feel like it's stripping your skin. My face is dry and often feels tight after cleansing but not with this. A great find.'

the science bit: Its formula aims to leave skin feeling supple rather than depleted after cleansing, and it includes ingredients that work to bind moisture into your skin. It can be rinsed off with water or wiped off with very soft tissue.

Lancôme Eau De Bienfait Clarte

£16 for 200ml

Despite the fact that this contains skin-buffing properties and is a 3-in-1 cleanser – acting as a refreshing toner and eye make-up remover as well as general skin cleanser, which is quite a lot of qualities for a humble cleanser – our testers really loved this product and felt it still met our criteria. In particular Anne (42) said, 'I was dubious that it could do all these things to my face, but I have to say it worked very well, and I liked not having to use a separate product to take my eye make-up off first. It saves time.'

the science bit: The formula includes a blend of vitamins plus extracts of skin-smoothing pineapple and papaya.

E'Spa Facial Foaming Cleanser £18.50 for 150ml

'This is a complete breakthrough for me and my sensitive skin,' said Heather (31), one of the people who tested this. 'A really lovely cleanser that smells gorgeous – I don't normally use scented products but I had no problems with this – and foams up and washes off easily. It's a joy to use in the mornings too because it wakes your skin – and you – up.'

the science bit: A foaming formula containing nourishing olive oil and honey, plus the natural cleansing agent coconut.

Clarins Cleansing Milk £13 for 200ml

Many of our testers said they go back to Clarins time and time again for cleansers because they trust the products to do what they say they will. 'I love the fragrance of Clarins products,' said Sara (31), 'it's familiar and reassuring, especially to come back to if you've been using something else.' Nina (37) also raved about this cleanser (she used the Alpine Herbs variant), 'It just does what it says it will do – takes your make-up off easily, and never causes irritation, and that's all I want.'

the science bit: The milks, which come in two variants – Alpine Herbs for dry/normal skin and Gentian for combination/oily skin – contain plant extracts and Clarins have gone to great lengths to develop a formula which won't disturb the skin's natural pH balance.

moisturisers

The world divides into two when it comes to moisturiser – those who wear it and those who don't! It's our mission to make sure those who *do* bother with it are using the best moisturiser possible, and to convert those who need it but don't use it.

Along with cleanser, moisturiser is the most valuable beauty product in your beauty regime. It's never too late to start using it and there are a hundred reasons why you should. Let's start with how your skin looks today: is it dull, patchy and a bit drawn? If so, the answer could be moisturiser. Next, how old does your skin look? If it appears to be ageing faster than you are the answer could be moisturiser again.

Face cream is a fundamental beauty requirement. It can't erase wrinkles, but it can help to preserve your skin and transform it in other ways, often in a very short space of time.

'all creams – from simple emollients to moisturisers with active anti-ageing ingredients – can be classed as anti-ageing because they all moisturise skin – a fundamental skin-preserving benefit'

The biggest problem moisturisers have are the high expectations we have of them. Because some creams make such outlandish claims (and several of our testers pointed this out to us – saying they 'never do what they promise') we tend to think that all moisturisers should do the same (take years off your skin), otherwise they are not worth using. But this is rubbish. Beauty is not just about having young, line-free skin – we all know this in our heart of hearts, and not every skin needs the latest hi-tech, all-action face cream: definitely not if it hasn't got any wrinkles on it! Sometimes the simplest and least expensive formulas can have the best effect on your skin. This is why it's so vital to get the right one.

One of our testers wrote 'it's time to lift the lid on what really works and why' on her questionnaire. We agree. You have come to the right place to find out.

Let the lid-lifting begin!

what makes a great moisturiser?

We get asked this a lot (along with how much you should pay for one), and the truth is that no one magic ingredient necessarily makes one cream better than another – nor does the claim that a moisturiser is anti-ageing. But a cream which has a sun protection factor (SPF) is a wiser investment than one which hasn't because it will prevent skin cancer and delay ageing. So the simple answer is that a good cream contains emollients and an SPF. Anything else is a bonus.

which moisturiser do I need?

This was something lots and lots of our testers asked: Vicky (40) rightly pointed out that 'there are so many variations – how do I know which cream is best for me?' Anna (33) asked, 'I'm so confused about the ingredients I should be looking for in a face cream – are some better for my skin than others? And are there any I should be avoiding at my age?' Yes to both questions and you will find out why on the following pages. Liza (39) simply wanted to know how many 'layers' of moisturiser to put on.

In a nutshell, face creams break down into three categories:

1. Moisturising – a simple emollient like cold cream.
2. Moisturising and protective – an emollient (which can be any consistency – such as serum, milk, emulsion, cream or gel) with a sun protective filter.
3. Moisturising, protective and anti-ageing – an emollient cream (of any consistency) containing a UV filter and ingredients which may have a de-ageing effect on your skin. It's worth noting though that a protective cream (number two on our list here) can also be described as anti-ageing because by moisturising and protecting your skin it is effectively slowing down ageing.

which ingredients should I look for?

One of our testers, Sally (50), said 'I'm confused by anti-wrinkle creams and I'm sure I'm not the only one. Which ingredients are best?' If you are at an age when you definitely need an active anti-ageing cream, these are the key ingredients to look for in a product (you will find a longer explanation on what they do in our Beauty Lexis on page 184):

1. Alpha hydroxy acids (AHAs or fruit acids) – a very popular ingredient in skin creams. AHAs, extracted from fruit, are non-abrasive exfoliators which make your skin smoother and softer.
2. Antioxidants – these can be plant extracts, vitamins or even tea extracts which have an anti-ageing benefit because they neutralise the effects of free radicals, the reactive molecules that age your skin, and which are generated by enemies such as ultraviolet (UV) light and cigarette smoke.
3. Vitamin A – also known as retin A and retinyl palmitate, is included in skin creams because it is said to be able to reverse the signs of age, particularly those caused by the sun.
4. Vitamin E – an antioxidant and a natural skin moisturiser.
5. Vitamin C – an antioxidant and it also encourages the production of collagen (the stuff under your skin which makes it firm and springy). This is why it is often included in anti-ageing creams.
6. Grape seed extract – is another strong antioxidant and the latest anti-ageing miracle 'discovery'. It is found in lots of new anti-ageing creams.

serum, cream, emulsion, oil, milk – which is the best type of moisturiser?

This depends on you, your skin and life style. Some people like the feel of a creamy moisturiser – especially at night; others prefer the lightness of a milk or emulsion (a cross between a cream and a gel); serums (lightweight gel-like moisturisers) claim to offer more intensive treatment, so are best to use as a boost when your skin is flagging (change of season usually); and oils are by nature more greasy (this was the main reason why they didn't generally get great reviews from our road testers). Don't let consistency and texture be your only guide to choosing a moisturiser though: formulas are so clever now that a lightweight milk can offer as intensive benefits as a rich cream. If you are not sure ask for a sample and try it for a couple of days *on your face* – the back of your hand is no indication to how a cream will feel on your face.

do you need night cream?

Lots of our testers wanted to know this when we sent them night creams asking, isn't my skin the same at night as it is during the day? Well, of course your skin *looks* the same when you are asleep, but under the surface its natural repair mechanisms are working overtime to compensate for the damage done during the day. What damage? Exposure to ultraviolet (UV) light mostly – and this is another difference between day and night creams: most day creams contain a UV filter to protect your skin and you obviously don't need this at night. Of course your skin can't mend all the damage, but the thinking is that a potent night cream can maximise the skin's repair system. And in answer to a question from one of our testers, Catherine (40) – 'Is it possible to buy a cream that can take ten years off me overnight?' Yes, it is: just read some of the reviews.

> ‘how much should you apply? We firmly believe that you should apply plenty of moisturiser – and don't stop at your jawline: your neck needs protective cream as much as your face does’

There is another reason why your skin might benefit from a night cream later in life. Less hormone activity in menopausal skin is more obvious in the morning because lymph slows down and your face is not so mobile at night. And some scientists think that if we use the right night creams we can prevent problems like early morning puffiness and 'pillow' creasing that are typical of menopausal skin.

when do you need anti-ageing moisturisers?

This was another big question for the people who took part in our survey. One of the biggest beauty *myths* is that we all need active anti-ageing moisturisers. This is total nonsense. All skins of all ages need a *proper* moisturiser, one which has a UV filter and lubricates skin (some beauty companies call this kind of moisturiser 'anti-ageing' because by keeping your skin hydrated and protected it is effectively staving off the ageing process); but until you get into your thirties you don't usually need to use creams with *active* anti-ageing ingredients (fruit acids, retin A, etc.) in them. We think AGE, not skin type, is the best guide to the sort of face creams you should be using, because it is one of the main factors that dictates how your skin develops. This hopefully answers one of our tester's questions – 'In which order should I tackle puffiness, wrinkles and sagging?'

> 'one of the biggest beauty myths is that we *all* need active anti-ageing creams'

Here is how your skin changes and matures in the different decades of your life – and what it needs:

teens to 20s – your skin is growing up; it's hormonal so a bit unreliable (especially during puberty), and can be greasy, spotty and sensitive, but it is also plump and firm.

you need: a simple unscented UV protective moisturiser (70 percent of a lifetime's sun damage can be done before the age of 16).

beauty scoop highly commends:

- Olay Complete Care (£7.49 for 50ml) – a simple vitamin-rich cream with (most importantly) an SPF of 15.
- Clinique Oil-Free Moisture Formula (£14.50 for 40ml) – a basic oil-free cream containing soothing aloe vera.
- Clarins Multi-Active Day Cream (£30 for 50ml) – developed to combat the drying and ageing effects of temperature swings like central heating and icy winds.
- Epure Be Matt (£15 for 50ml) – developed for teenagers with oily skin, this cream contains a nylon polymer which soaks up surface oil like a sponge.

you don't need: stimulating moisturisers with active anti-ageing ingredients like fruit acids (hydroxy acids) in them or creams which claim to control sebum and oil production – different to those which only claim to keep the surface matt.

30s to 40s – cell renewal slows down, lines appear near your eyes. Stress makes your skin look dull and 'pinched', and your blood vessels dilate causing broken veins. Skin blooms when you are pregnant, but you may also experience hyper-pigmentation problems (when it seems to go a bit patchy), and after childbirth skin loses a lot of suppleness and expression lines form more quickly.

you need: of all the different age-groups that tried products for us, this was the one most confused about the creams they need. So here is the answer: you need creams which aim to promote collagen production in your skin – look for those containing ingredients such as vitamin C as they can help to keep skin springy; creams which make your skin smoother and more radiant; active anti-ageing lip cream or balm.

beauty scoop highly commends:

- Boots Time Delay Repair Day Moisturise (£10 for 50ml) – contains lifting and collagen-strengthening agents like white lupin extract, and improves skin's natural lipid barrier so it retains moisture.
- Lancôme Vinefit Complete Energising Moisturiser SPF15 (£26 for 50ml) – is based on the antioxidant (anti-ageing) benefits of grapes and polyphenols.
- Re Vive Lip & Perioral Renewal Cream (£78 for 15ml) – contains an epidermal growth factor which repairs damage caused by dryness and builds up resistance to chapping. (We think this is the 'Crème de la Mer' of lip creams.)

you don't need: really heavy day or night creams.

50s plus – more of the same, plus the menopause can have an impact on your skin, causing spots, accelerating collagen loss – which makes your skin less elastic and thinner (but thicker around your pores which is why they look more open and pronounced) – and triggering hyper-pigmentation. When menopause is over a slowdown in oestrogen production reduces sebum output, so your skin becomes much drier.

you need: rich but lightweight day and night-time creams with active anti-ageing benefits which won't clog your pores but will give your skin the support it needs; active anti-ageing lip cream or balm.

beauty scoop highly commends:

- Clarins Super Restorative Serum (£62 for 30ml) – contains pueraria lobata (ivy extract) and pelvetia (seaweed) which have firming and elasticising benefits.
- Yves Saint Laurent Age Expert Crème (£35 for 30ml) – a pioneering cream which contains a synthetic form of DHEA, known as the 'molecule of youthfulness' because it helps to keep skin young and plump.
- Gatineau Electelle Beautifying Lip Care (£17.75 for 15ml) – a treatment lip cream (not balm) which moisturises and contains protein microspheres to volumise lips.
- B Kamins Menopause Skin Cream (£82 for 45gm) – a hi-tech formula which aims to combat the big changes skin goes through before, during and after menopause.
- Guerlain Issima Substantific Day Crème (£45 for 30ml) – a supremely nourishing but lightweight cream for dry skin with a SPF of 10.

you don't need: oil-controlling moisturisers, soap (it is far too drying), and water-based creams (not hydrating enough).

Five good reasons to bin your moisturiser and buy another one:

1. It stings or makes your skin go red and blotchy: it may have ingredients in it that your skin doesn't like (you will find a list of properties that commonly irritate in our Beauty Lexis on page 187), be over-fragranced or past its sell-by date.
2. It hasn't got a proper broadspectrum sun filter: one of our testers, Janey (45), posed the question, 'If wearing an SPF at all times is so important, why isn't it added to all products?' Obviously you don't need sunscreen in a night cream but other products – such as intensive serums – don't contain a filter because it might compromise the product's active ingredients and overall performance. Also, not everybody wants to wear a cream with a sunscreen in it everyday – some believe it will weaken their skin's natural defence mechanism – so the beauty business is giving us a choice (although admittedly it is hard to find a day cream now without a sun filter in it). If the day cream you like doesn't have one, and you want UV defense, wear protective foundation over the top.
3. It makes your skin feel greasy: there is no excuse for this – the only exception is a night-time facial oil, but the decent ones tend to absorb very well.

4. It smells vile (something which usually becomes most obvious when you get into bed with it on): it is probably past its sell-by date.
5. It is past its sell-by date: all beauty products contain chemical preservatives (even 'natural' ones), but most products still have a shelf-life, albeit a varying one, so it is worth checking this when you buy the product.

are expensive moisturisers better than cheap ones?

Not necessarily. Kate admits she is happy to spend money on face creams, but you don't have to splash out to get a good one because the effects depend on you, your skin and its needs. Some of our testers said that the best moisturisers they have used have been the cheaper ones; others gave expensive serums the thumbs down because they dehydrated their skin. Expensive products can cost more because:

- **time**: if it is a pioneering formula – which expensive creams often are – more research may have gone into them (some creams take a decade to develop which is a long time for world-class scientists to be in a lab). Interestingly though, some premium brands make products for cheaper brands and vice versa: Estée Lauder own many brands, including Stila, Jo Malone, Bobbi Brown, Aveda and Crème de la Mer, all of which vary in price; Chanel make Bourjois' cheap and cheerful make-up; and L'Oreal – who sell fairly competitive products – also make Lancôme and Helena Rubinstein's more expensive cosmetics.
- **quality**: they *may* contain better quality ingredients like liposomes or silk pigments that help products glide more smoothly onto your skin, feel better once there and, arguably, perform better.
- **animal tests**: many beauty houses including Revlon, Shiseido, Estee Lauder and L'Oréal invest millions into developing alternative animal tests.
- **packaging**: there is no getting away from it, the bottle and box often take the lion's share of the costs involved in developing a product.
- **psychology**: because many people think all expensive products are more effective than cheaper ones, manufacturers price their products accordingly. A couple of our testers said they thought manufacturers 'also tried to blind consumers with science to make the product sound more appealing'. Which is a good point.

Remember these tips next time you are about to spend an arm and a leg on a new moisturiser.

shopping for moisturisers

Before you head for the shops or flash your cash:

1. Do your research and decide which moisturiser your skin actually *needs* – rather than just going for the latest one you have read about in the magazines or seen advertised on TV. Don't be taken in by the images that go with face cream adverts: remember that the models look the way they do because they are groomed by world-class make-up artists, photographed in very flattering light and then air-brushed to perfection – even though they are probably not even at an age where they need the class of cream you are looking for.
2. Ask for a sample to take home (especially if you are making an investment). The beauty counters should oblige, but if not and you have got access to the internet visit www.QVC.co.uk – the shopping channel QVC's website. They sell most of the popular brands and have a unique returns policy if you buy a product from them and decide you don't like it: *you can send it back* – even if you have opened the pot and stuck your fingers in it. Now that is what we call service!
3. Decide how much you want to spend: the results from our survey showed that you can find excellent moisturisers (anti-ageing or otherwise) from brands across the board, so you don't have to take out a second mortgage to buy a decent one. Although most expensive creams cost more for the reasons we have highlighted, there is also hype to consider: some 'super-premium creams' are marketed to make you *think* they are the best simply because they cost an extortionate amount of money. It is worth being aware of this.

... moisturisers we rate:

Julia Neal's Yard Remedies Organic Violet Day Cream (£14.75 for 30ml) and Rose & Almond Night Cream (£15.75 for 30ml): 'Together, these two made the most visible difference to my skin that I've seen in a long while. In winter though I like Sisley Confort Extreme Night Skin Care (£69 for 50ml) – it's really soothing, and great for dry skin. And despite the price, I buy Guerlain Issima Midnight Secret (£51 for 30ml) – it's my skin saviour.'

Kate La Prairie Extract of Caviar Firming Complex (£76 for 30ml): 'I'm a total snob about moisturiser – I'll pay over the odds for it – and this cream is the reason why. It proved to me that moisturiser really can have a visible impact on your skin. I first used it ten years ago and am still writing about it now – all those testers who told us that their dream cream would be one which instantly makes them look ten years younger should try it. I also love Sisley Ecological Compound (£46 for 50ml), it's very light and it smells heavenly.'

the best moisturisers

the mission: To find you the most effective and user-friendly day and night-time face creams on the market.

the criteria Our testers judged the day creams they tried on their ability to deliver the promises they made – to hydrate skin, make it firmer, smoother, and perhaps more even-toned. They also judged the creams on their wearability – how comfortable they are on the skin; how easy they are to apply, their feel (i.e. lightweight and non-greasy) and smell.

the 9 best day creams

Estée Lauder Daywear Plus Moisturiser £26 for 50ml

Linda (42) said, 'I'll be honest, I was a bit disappointed when you sent me this – it just looks so boring. But I've been using it now for just over five weeks and it's made a real difference to my skin. The change is mostly in its texture. It's plumper and suppler. But it makes the world of difference to me. I think this is a really good cream.' Victoria (32) said: 'It made my skin feel lovely and fresh', and Jane (41) said: 'My skin felt smoother as soon as I put it on. The results are still visible and my skin looks firmer after a few hours'.

the science bit: The formula contains eight different antioxidants, including grape seed extract, south African red tea (that is rooibos to anyone who is familiar with the strong cuppa), resveretrol and rosemary, plus hyaluronic acid, a big skin moisturiser and an SPF of 15.

Avon Anew Pure O2 Cream SPF15 £15 for 50ml

'Since you sent me this I've got my best friend Lynne to buy one too because I think it's such a good cream,' wrote Shirley (50). 'And she loves it too. It says it puts oxygen into your skin which sounds a bit strange, but it must be a good thing because my skin is blooming.' Another tester, Chris (44) wrote 'great value for money'.

the science bit: The formula contains Avon's special anti-ageing complex – rejuiv-technology, which regenerates and moisturises skin, and improves clarity.

Nivea Q10 Anti-Wrinkle Day Cream

£9.69 for 50ml

'The packaging isn't up to much,' wrote Jenny (30), 'but I can't fault the cream. My partner says I look like I've had a transplant – sorry, face-lift! I'm really impressed by it. Is there a cleanser to go with it?' Dee (58) wrote, 'I've always rated Nivea. I think the cheaper brands are just as good as the pricey ones. This cream's a gem.'

the science bit: Q10 is a co-enzyme which is found naturally in our bodies and which Nivea have added to this cream to regenerate skin and diminish lines.

No7 Daily V Essential Moisture Cream

£7.90 for 100ml

All the testers who tried this gave it full marks, except one, who felt it was too thick and 'suffocating' on her skin. Kate (42) said 'good texture. It conditioned my skin and it's a great cheaper option.' Kerry-Ann (32) said, 'My mother and auntie swear by No7 and I've always turned my nose up at it a bit because I think it's a bit old-ladyish. But this cream is FAB. Who would have thought such a well-priced cream could have made my skin so much softer and more radiant? Not me!'

the science bit: Key ingredients are vitamin E, the antioxidant and super-hydrator, rosewater (which gives it a lovely gentle scent) and elderflower to replenish and soothe skin.

Elizabeth Arden Ceramide Plump Perfect Moisture Cream SPF15

£40 for 50ml

'I was SO excited when this arrived in the post,' Liz (58) – one of the women who tried this – told us. 'My husband said to calm down because he thinks all creams are the same and just sell a load of hype to us women. But I've been using it daily now for nearly six weeks and I've been converted – not just to this cream but to using face cream full stop. The main difference is my skin's suppleness, something I noticed had changed since the menopause. It's like it was five or ten years ago. Thank you.'

the science bit: The main ingredient is argirelene, a complex of six amino acids which plumps up lines and makes them look less obvious.

Crème De La Mer

£75 for 30ml

A couple of our testers insisted that this cream is 'not worth the hype'. But we could not ignore the praise that has been heaped on this cream by editors and friends who have tried it. Annabel (39) is a convert: 'Unfortunately someone let me try some of their's once,' she told us, 'and there was no going back. It was a pivotal skin care moment for me.' Deirdre (57) said, 'I've never dared tell my husband how much it costs, but I think it's worth every penny.' Those are just two of the many positive verbal testimonials we have had. This cream needs to be tried to be believed.

the science bit: the core of this formula is a 'miracle broth', created with sea kelp that is put through a bio-fermentation process.

Ponds Cold Cream

£3.39 for 100ml

So many of the people who took part in our survey said they thought this was one of the best face creams you can buy yet is completely overshadowed by products which claim to give you the earth and actually do very little. 'There's a reason it's been around for so long,' said Angela (54), 'it's reliable. You know it's going to nourish your skin without irritating it, and it absorbs well if you apply a thin layer.' 'It went off the market for a while,' wrote Sue (40), 'but I've been told it's back. I can't believe they even thought they needed to take it away in the first place!'

the science bit: The formula is enriched with emollients and skin conditioners.

Eau Thermale Avène Hydrance Optimale Light Hydrating Cream

£12.50 for 40ml

Sammy (23) and Maureen (67) both loved this cream for its simplicity: 'Sometimes I think beauty has forgotton about women who just want a very simple moisturiser – not an all-singing-all-dancing anti-ageing cream,' said Maureen. 'But there are lots of us out there! I like a light, gentle cream because I've got sensitive skin. This suits me perfectly; I'll probably move on from the cold cream I've been using now.'

the science bit: The key ingredients are thermal spring water from Avene in France, and moisture-binders to maintain the skin's natural barrier.

Jurlique Herbal Recovery Gel

£42.50 for 30ml

The original 'facelift in a bottle', this refreshing gel is amazingly good at making your skin look rested and making it feel firmer and plumper. 'I put it on in the evening before going out and the effects were so good I was tempted not to bother with makeup', said Cathy (58). She wore it under her moisturiser the following day and found that it was just as powerful. 'Every so often you come across these little beauty miracles and you can't believe you've lived without them', said Cathy, 'and this is one of them!'

the science bit: super-concentrated, the gel is crammed with botanical antioxidant extracts like echinacea, green tea, vitamin E and grape seed.

the 10 best night treatments

Vichy Novadiol Night
£17.50 for 50ml

Ruth (52) was one of the testers who thought this cream performed well. 'My skin has taken a turn for the worse over the past couple of years. In the mornings it's puffy – especially under my eyes – and at night it's just flat and pinched,' she told us. 'But I've got on well with this. It's specially good at brightening your skin up.' Ruth didn't notice much difference in her puffiness, but Faye (58) did. She told us, 'I just seem to look less crumpled in the morning – it's as if my skin has been ironed. I liked the smell of it too – it's a sort of mild cut grass scent.'

the science bit: The key ingredients are plant growth regulators and phyto-oestrogens which increase collagen production, caffeine – a skin decongestant – and gatuline, which boosts cell renewal.

Neutrogena Regenerating Night Cream
£6.99 for 50ml

'This is real no-fuss stuff – is that why you sent it to me?' asked Tonie (31), a friend who admits she doesn't have time for (her words) 'all that beauty flannel'. As it turns out, it was the right one to send her because she has since asked where she can get some more: 'It's just so nice to have soft, supple skin,' she said. 'I always thought you had to use those heavy duty cold creams to make your skin feel nice.'

the science bit: The formula contains active cell-regenerating properties and glycerine to give skin a hydrating boost.

Aromatherapy Associates Rose & Frankincense Facial Oil
£25 for 15ml

Facial oils didn't do too well in our road tests on the whole, but this one – blended by the UK's leading aromatherapists (in our opinion) – was one of the two that came out well, with several testers saying they were 'delighted' to have discovered it because it seemed to suit their skin better than cream. 'It's not too greasy because most of it's absorbed, but it is greasier than a cream, there is no getting away from that,' said June (49). 'It's done wonders for my skin's suppleness and it smells gorgeous.'

the science bit: As its name suggests, the oil is a blend of two main essential oils – rose and frankincense – which have nourishing and reparative benefits.

Helena Rubinstein Collagenist Night Cream
£50 for 50ml

This is a serious action anti-ageing cream which mainly targets skin elasticity and plumpness. Maxine (52) saw the greatest difference in her neck: 'It improved the skin there enormously,' she said, 'and its performance all round was very good.' Tania (31) has been thinking about Botox, so we got her to try this cream first, and she was impressed. 'The lines from my nose to my mouth do look better,' she said.

the science bit: The formula's two active agents – cytovitine (a yeast extract) and phytokine (derived from soya protein) – are said to stimulate collagen synthesis in the skin.

No7 Daily V Nourishing Night Cream £8.95 for 100ml

A very decent night cream that scored 10/10 for Leah (55) who said, 'It's not scented – I was glad about that because my skin is sensitive, and it felt comfortable to wear. I've noticed my skin is brighter and fresher looking, so it does live up to its claims.'

the science bit: the key ingredients are skin-calming camomile, reviving watercress extract, and the super-hydrators vitamin E and pro-vitamin B5.

Amanda Lacey Camellia Oil £34.50 for 30ml

Top facialist Amanda Lacey specially developed this facial oil to be user-friendly – in other words, to absorb without leaving an oily residue on your skin. 'It's a lovely rich golden oil, and the minute I started rubbing it in my skin seemed to thank me,' remarked Lauren (34); 'I've never used an oil before – this is a first for me,' wrote Hilary (44), 'I've always been put off by the grease factor. But I was amazed at how much of it disappeared into my skin.' Both testers remarked on its 'divine' scent, too.

the science bit: Amanda is a perfectionist when it comes to her products, so the ingredients you find in this oil – camellia oil, vitamin E and essential oils of rose, roman camomile, rosemary and silver fir – are the finest quality.

Elemis Absolute Night Cream £29 for 50ml

'What a nice way to go to bed,' said one of our testers Emma (32) after sampling this cream. 'It's got a really lovely smell of jasmine and orange. It's very nourishing too, but not horrible and heavy – I can't bear that feeling when you go to bed and your face sticks to the pillow. My skin is so much softer and more pingy.'

the science bit: Available in two formulas, the cream for normal/dry skin includes lavender, blackcurrant, sandalwood and comfrey to repair, hydrate and energise skin; and the one for normal/combination skin includes jasmine absolute, ylang ylang, camomile, cardamom and orange to hydrate and balance.

RoC Soya Unifying Nourishing Cream Night

£19.95 for 50ml

RoC products were very popular with our testers, and one of the reasons for this – apart from the fact that they feel they offer sophisticated skincare at an affordable price – is that the products are not as heavily marketed as some brands: lots and lots of our testers said that pushy marketing was a total turn-off. 'I don't want to pay the earth for a moisturiser,' said Emma (39), who was happy to test this product for us because she is a RoC fan anyway. 'I still have some pigmentation patches on my face,' she told us, a month after starting treatment, 'but the one on the left hand side of my forehead – a leftover from my last pregnancy – is definitely less obvious. I'm really excited about it.'

the science bit: RoC have applied active soya technology – a special patent they have developed – to this cream to help reduce the appearance of dark spots and boost skin radiance.

exfoliators

Skin feels so great after it's been exfoliated, doesn't it? Soft, smooth, warm and glowing. It wasn't always like this though. About thirty years ago, abrasive exfoliators didn't even exist. The job was done by alcoholic toners and skin suffered the drying and irritating consequences of having its top layer burned off with the stuff.

'when not to exfoliate: when your skin is sensitive, paper thin (a side effect of aged skin), has rosacea or a disorder like psoriasis, eczema or dermatitis'

Then the beauty scientists brought us mechanical scrubs – abrasive creams or gels with particles such as almond pits in them that physically buffed off dead skin cells. Afterwards we got scruffing pads and puffs – abrasive bits of foam that made skin soft, yes, but often very angry and irritated too.

And now you can buy peels that dry like a mask on your skin and lift off dead skin cells when you roll them off, creams which contain alpha hydroxy acids (AHAs) that buff skin chemically instead of physically abrading it – so doing all the work without you having to lift a finger – and scrubs with buffing particles as fine as marble dust.

Which is best? Read on to find out what our criteria is for a good (and bad) skin buffer – and which ones came out on top in our road tests.

why bother exfoliating?

So you get softer skin – what else? A lot! Exfoliating has the following benefits for all skin types:

- It removes excess or built-up dead skin cells on the surface of your skin immediately makes it look brighter and over time improves its texture because healthier, younger cells are able to come to the surface.
- It helps to keep pores uncongested (by shifting dead skin) which means you get less spots.
- It enhances your circulation, so fresh blood – rich in nutrients – rises up to the surface of your skin to feed the cells and make skin pink and plump.
- It allows moisturiser to penetrate skin more easily because there are fewer dried-up dead skin cells in the way blocking absorption.

what makes a great exfoliator?

- A high concentration of *extremely fine* buffing particles – think ground marble or baking soda. Exfoliators which have a smattering of big buffing grains (like ground nut shells or soft 'beads') are a complete waste of time.
- A water-soluble cream or gel that can be washed-off (but we still think it's a good idea to use a hot flannel to wipe off the residue).
- Quick drying so it can be rolled off easily with your fingers and doesn't leave a 'rubbery' residue on your skin.
- No scent – at least nothing perceptible – and ideally no 'minty' ingredients like peppermint, menthol, eucalyptus or alcohol as these can all irritate your face.

what's best – mechanical or chemical scrubs?

The jury is out on whether it's best to use a gritty exfoliator which removes dead skin mechanically by abrasion, a peel-off one or a non-abrasive chemical one which contains fruit acids. These sound quite scary but fruit (alpha and beta hydroxy) acids are popular ingredients in exfoliators, cleansers and moisturisers now, and work on a deeper level than regular scrubs. You can find out more about hydroxy acids in the chapter on moisturisers (see page 18), but if you're a serious beauty junkie and want to know about all the latest advances, the difference between them is that *beta* hydroxy acids can cut through sebum so they work on a deeper level than *alpha* hydroxy acids.

shopping for exfoliators

Before you head for the shops or flash your cash:

1. Make sure the exfoliator you want has a dense filling of the finest buffing grains you can find – there is nothing more frustrating than trying to scrub your skin with an exfoliator that doesn't have enough grains in it.
2. Decide what type of exfoliator you want – foam-up and wash-off, cream or peel? It depends on your life style and skin type – a wash-off one could make dry skin even thirstier, but you might not have the time to use a peel-off one.
3. Decide how much you want to spend: our testers found that exfoliators in the mid-to-premium ranges worked best.

... exfoliators we rate:

Julia 'A flannel! It seems to do the job just fine for me – and it's a lot more gentle than many abrasive skin-buffers.'

Kate 'Ditto. And they seem to work better the older, harder and more knobbly they get.'

the 5 best face exfoliators

the mission To find you the most effective and user-friendly face exfoliators on the market.

the criteria Our testers judged the face exfoliators they tried on their ability to improve skin softness and radiance, on the density of their buffing grains (the higher the better), on their ability to leave skin supple – not dry and taut – and their fragrance. The results of our test showed that you do have to pay a bit more for a good exfoliator as the ones that made our top-of-the-pile list were those in the mid and top end of the market.

Estée Lauder Idealist Micro-D Deep Thermal Refinisher

£29 for 75ml

A pale cream that doesn't look like it's going to do much until you start massaging it into your skin and then it starts to warm up and feel gritty. A good exfoliator will give instant results – definitely the case with this one. One of our testers said her skin felt 'softer, smoother and better toned', which is an added bonus. Pamela (62) said, 'I'd never spend this much on any beauty product – let alone an exfoliator – normally, but I'm so impressed by it I've been telling all my friends to get it.'

the science bit: It includes not one but three different types of micro-surfacing spheres (beauty speak for 'exfoliating grains') – microcrystalline, jade and bamboo extracts – because Lauder believes this gives a more intense cleanse. The idea behind the warming sensation, created by an ingredient called calcium chloride, is that it enhances your skin's natural cleansing processes.

Darphin Mild Aroma Peeling

£22 for 50ml

Of all the peel-off exfoliators you tried this was the one our testers liked best. 'I was amazed at how well it worked,' said Imogen (35). 'I didn't think it would have the same smoothing effects or oomph as grains, but it was ten times better than any grainy exfoliator I've used in the past, and it doesn't make your skin dry.' Sasha (28) pointed out that it 'would be ideal for anyone with sensitive skin because it's not abrasive'. Jo (39) liked it, but recommends peeling it off over a sink 'otherwise your bathroom gets covered in lots of annoying bits of dead skin and dry exfoliator'. Nice.

the science bit: Ideal for sensitive skins, this exfoliator doesn't use grit to shift dead skin; it dries on your skin and when you rub it off it takes the dead cells with it. It does contain lemon and pineapple though, so there is some fruit (alpha hydroxy) acid action going on too.

Fresh Rich Face Wash

£27.50 for 105gm

Lisa (37) hasn't used an exfoliator in the past because she says her skin is sensitive and buffing it makes it more vulnerable – 'It's as if I'm opening it up to the elements,' she said. She had never heard of Fresh products before she agreed to try this buffer for us, and is so impressed by it she admits she is now using it to cleanse and exfoliate every week. 'I haven't had any reaction to it which I'm delighted about,' she says, 'and I'm also thrilled with the way my skin looks. Thank you!'

the science bit: The formula includes lots of super-fine rich starch and powdered rice bran to give skin a thorough but very soft polish.

Caudalie Gentle Buffing Cream

£15 for 50ml

'The grains are so small in this cream you can't even feel them scrubbing your skin,' said Christina (30). 'So it's not harsh on your skin – you could probably get away with using it quite regularly – but it's still effective. My skin had a real sparkle to it.'

the science bit: The formula is packed with interesting ingredients such as organic licorice, coriander, French honey and grape seed extracts – a feature of all Caudalie's beauty products, and noted for its ability to neutralise free radicals, the reactive molecules that age our skin.

Bliss Spa Sleeping Peel Micro Exfoliating Mask

£38 for 1oz

'Are there any exfoliators out there that do the work for you while you sleep?' asked a couple of our (very lazy) testers. Yes, and Sophie (28) tried it for us having admitted she 'can't really be bothered with exfoliating'. She was more impressed by the results than the actual product though. 'It's just a mask-type exfoliator which you put on and leave to do all the hard work for you – you barely even have to massage it into your skin. It needs five minutes on your face and then you rinse it off. Seriously low fuss-factor. But the results were really, really good. My skin looked much brighter. I don't know why anyone would want to use an ordinary exfoliator.'

the science bit: This is a clay-based mask which targets blackheads and pores – drawing impurities out of them, and has a natural exfoliative effect on skin.

masks

We know from our survey that most of you don't have time for masks. None of the people who took part in our research even mentioned the word mask when they described their skin care routines. But lots of them (mainly those with children) said that because they did not have time for facials they would like an intensive treatment they could use at night and which would take years off their faces by morning.

> 'milk of magnesium – that awful liquid magnesium you take for constipation – makes a good anti-inflammatory mask for spotty zones'

This is exactly what a decent mask can do for you: the best ones transform your skin and raise your spirits – something we all need every now and then.

So how do you go about finding a good one?

Well, the first thing to do is to decide what you want out of a face mask. Think about what your skin needs – a radiance boost perhaps, a deep-pore cleanse around your nose and chin, or a good long drink: something skin often needs in winter.

Next, you need to work out when you are going to use the mask. In an ideal world you should put it on and relax – not run around clearing up, unloading the dish-washer, replying to emails or doing the Hoovering! Obviously this is out of the question for most of us in the day, but it is usually possible to find time in the evening – when you are comatose in front of the TV or lying in the bath – to treat your skin with a mask.

Masks are pretty uncomplicated beauty products – and they are optional: your skin doesn't need them like it needs moisturiser. But if you are going to buy one try to use it regularly (i.e. every week) so your skin gets the maximum benefits.

'masks are a great way to give your skin an instant hit, but don't forget – some of the best skin boosters are actually free: sleep and fresh air'

how to maximise the effects of a mask

1. Exfoliate your skin first with a fine-grained scrub to make your skin more receptive to treatment; rinse with warm water and pat skin dry.
2. Apply the face mask – either all over your face (excluding the eye and mouth area) or just to the parts where it is needed: deep-cleansing masks are usually needed most on oil-prone zones like your chin and nose, while hydrating masks are required on cheeks and jawline, where skin gets thirstier.
3. RELAX: put some hand cream on, have a cup of tea or read the newspaper.
4. Remove the mask – either by splashing your face with water and removing the residue with a face cloth (just as you would water-soluble cleanser), or by wiping it off with a cottonwool pad. Apply moisturiser if needed.

what makes a great face mask?

One which doesn't make too many claims! We think masks which offer too many benefits compromise themselves by trying to achieve too much. The best masks make believable claims – for example, to deep-cleanse, hydrate or firm – not claim to do all these things, plus walk the dog, cook supper and put the children to bed.

shopping for masks

Before you head for the shops or flash your cash:

1. Work out what kind of mask you need – one to deep-cleanse your skin, firm or hydrate it. This helps to narrow down the choice.
2. Consider your life style: some masks are specially developed to work fast or overnight so your skin gets the benefits and you can get on with living.
3. Decide how much you want to spend: none of the masks our testers rated are particularly cheap. But don't forget, a mask isn't like a moisturiser in that you need to apply it daily – once a week or fortnight is usually enough to reap the benefits – so a 50ml tube should last at least six months.

... face masks we rate:

Julia No7 Hydra Boost Mask (£12 for 100ml): 'As I've got older I've found that my skin has got drier so I mostly use moisturising masks, and when I've got time I tend to go back to this one. It's a lovely smelling pink cream that doesn't need to be on for long to do the job well.'

Kate 'I've never found a mask that works better than the one I make myself. It's a beaten egg mixed with a teaspoon of olive oil that you slosh all over your face with cotton buds saturated in the stuff and rinse off when it dries. Your skin looks amazing and you don't need moisturiser afterwards because your skin feels supple with a bit of a healthy sheen.'

the 8 best face masks

the mission To find you the most effective and user-friendly face masks on the market.

the criteria Our testers judged the face masks they tried on their ability to hydrate the skin, deep-cleanse it, improve radiance, tone and relaxation – we wanted to know if any masks could *really* make your faces look rested. They also judged the masks on efficacy, speed of results and that all-important feature – smell.

Wu Morning! Mask

£23.50 for 50ml

'Luckily I'd read about this product before I offered to try it for you,' wrote Paula (36), 'otherwise I'd have had a fit and tried to wash it off very quickly! It's really unbelievable – exactly as people have described it. You feel like you have stuck your face in a bucket of ice, and the effects are fantastic. Much firmer skin. And talk about a good hangover cure!' Shirley (56) was equally surprised: 'I didn't think you could buy products like this,' she said. 'It's so powerful, it blows your head off when you've got it on and afterwards your skin gets this chilly glow. Very invigorating.'

the science bit: The magic ingredients are herbs that have a powerful astringent and cooling effect on skin.

Ella Baché Beautifying Mask

£15.95 for 75ml

Helen (37) said, 'My hackles went up when I got this mask because I thought its "beautifying" claims were a bit dubious.' Luckily she didn't back out and wrote, 'I was surprised because it *did* give me a glowing complexion – which is certainly more beautiful than my usual washed-out look. My lines didn't spring out and hit me when I looked at my face and it seemed less drawn. Excellent product, no detectible smell.'

the science bit: Forget the claims to 'refine' pores, this clay-based mask works extremely well to smooth and calm skin – it's got camomile and allantoin in it. Apply a generous layer (and you can put it near to your eyes) and leave it on for at least ten minutes.

The Lift

£79 for 10 treatments

Tricky one this to test because we know how uncomfortable it is – and how effective if you hang on in there. But we could not guarantee our testers' patience. Those who stuck it out though agreed that efficacy was not its biggest virtue but that the end result outweighed this negative. 'Wow! Who invented *this*?' asked Trudy (46). 'They deserve a medal. It works so well you can't believe it.' 'It itches and it's a total pfaff,' wrote Margaret (54), 'but a total miracle too. I can honestly say it took ten years off me – no, make that fifteen! And people commented on my skin. Is this what they mean by 'suffering' for beauty? I'd still use it if it smelled like manure.'

the science bit: The main magic 'tightening' and 'lifting' ingredient is corn starch, but it also contains papaya (a natural exfoliator) which enhances skin smoothness, and firming algae extract.

Christian Breton Instant Radiance Express Radiance Mask

£13.50 for 50ml

Two things worked in this product's favour as far as our testers were concerned: speed and vitality. 'It's a real workhorse,' said Lottie (39), 'it's quick, it's got a light and pleasant scent, and there's no need to wash it off – you just let it sink into your skin and it makes it look so much more alive. Does that sound a bit mad?' Emma (40), another tester, went so far as to say that 'my wrinkles are less apparent'.

the science bit: The secret to this creamy pink mask is crushed pearls – they give skin an amazingly natural radiance and luminosity.

Chanel Continuous Hydrating Mask £19.50 for 75ml

A comforting thirst-quencher this one, so ideal for skins that are dry or more mature. 'At my age my skin needs all the help it can get,' said Jo (45). 'This mask really helped – mainly because it made my skin so soft and look a bit plumped-up. It's creamy, luxurious, smells nice and fresh and it's something I'd be prepared to buy again. I don't think it's a bad price for Chanel. And it made me feel a bit spoilt.'

the science bit: The magic plumping and softening ingredients are D panthenol and allantoin, while vitamin E feeds and plumps-up skin.

Bioré Self Heating Mask £7.50 for 6 sachets

The best of the cheapie masks. Sally (22) said, 'I love the way it warms up – it really feels as if it's doing a proper job at dejunking my skin. There's no messy mud to worry about either.' And Helen (37) tried it and was so pleased with it she got her mother and sister-in-law to give it a go, too. They all reported good results: cleaner, firmer skin. 'It's perfect for priming your skin before a night out,' said Sally.

the science bit: The mask's clay content releases heat when it comes into contact with water – a little chemical change takes place if you like – and within about a minute it warms up to about 39 to 40 degrees C. The idea is that this facilitates the skin's natural cleansing system, so you get a deeper pore clean.

Elizabeth Arden Peel & Reveal Revitalizing Treatment £24 for 50ml

'This felt like a salon treatment you can actually do at home without getting in a terrible mess,' said Josie (34). 'The only drawback is the wait. You paint a thin layer onto your face with the brush you get and then have to leave it there for about half an hour before peeling it off. It is worth the bother though. My skin looked clearer and felt softer. It really felt like a special treat.'

the science bit: A classic chemical exfoliating mask, it contains beta and alpha hydroxy acids (BHAs and AHAs) and sugar extracts to buff and revitalise the skin, plus soothing and moisturising aloe vera.

Christian Dior Masque Stretch Firming Energy Mask £19.50 for 50ml

'Great name this! No real stretchy business went on with the actual mask,' wrote Lauren (34). 'But it did have a sort of firming feel as soon as I put it on my face, as if it was holding itself in place. It's hard to describe. It lifted my face and made me look much less tired. It's a nice-looking pale aqua cream and it smells divine – a mixture of grapefruit, musk, clove and basil. I'd buy it for its smell alone actually.'

the science bit: This mask uses the latest time-defying ingredient – grape seeds (which are said to have a beneficial astringent effect), wheat peptides (thought to help firm skin), and beech bud which has an energising effect on skin.

Kiehl's Soothing Gel Masque £17.50 for 50ml

Toni (31), who works in front of a computer all day, tried this out for us and said that her skin 'literally sucked it up like a Hoover. It must have been very thirsty! Perhaps it's all that computer abuse. But it's very refreshing. I left it on for about 20 minutes and it certainly made my skin look more rested - less run down'.

the science bit: This honey-coloured mask contains camomile and dandelion because they have potent soothing properties, plus the well-used antioxidant green tea extract.

lip treatments

Like your eyes, your lips are in a vulnerable position and need all the help they can get to keep them – and the skin around them – healthy and plump.

The skin that covers your lips has no melanin and is very thin, so blood vessels show through them and this is why they are typically red. They have no sweat glands and few sebaceous glands, so their only natural protection is saliva – a double-edged sword because the constant evaporation of moisture on lips leads to chapping.

> 'can you get addicted to balm? Not unless you use one that irritates your lips and makes them dry'

Your lips are always moving (again like your eyes), and because they are so exposed, they are prone to minor problems like cold sores and major ones like cancer. In fact, research done in the US has shown that men suffer from pre-malignant lesions and cancer of the lower lip more than women because we wear lipstick which gives us some level of physical protection from ultraviolet (UV) light.

The conclusion is then that your lips need daily lubrication and protection – something that can be provided by lip balms and some lipsticks and glosses.

What makes a good lip balm?

1. Emolliency: the more emollient they are the better. Shea and cocoa butter, and oils like castor, safflower, almond and vegetable are all good lip lubricants but however emollient, a good lip balm should be stable and not too sticky.
2. Good absorption: balm should be easily absorbed by your lips – lots just sit on top of your lips and your hair gets stuck to them. Arrgh!
3. Protection: daytime balms should contain a sun protection factor (SPF) if you are not wearing a protective lip-colour on top.

NB: some balms claim to be 'medicated', which usually means they contain ingredients like camphor, peppermint and menthol, but this doesn't necessarily make them any better than any other lip balm.

how smoking affects your lips

We have said it before in the book – and we will probably say it again: don't smoke! Apart from the health implications, cigarette smoke is almost as ageing for your skin as ultraviolet (UV) light. It contains billions of free radicals, the molecules that age skin, and the smoke only needs to touch your skin to wreak havoc. What's more, every time you purse your lips to drag on a cigarette the elasticity around your mouth is pressurised, which means lines form faster and your lip-line gets damaged. Smokers often find that they even get an indentation on their top lip from where they habitually put the cigarette. Pathetically, that was the turning point for Kate. GIVE IT UP.

how to rescue chapped lips

Because your lips don't have any natural lubrication they crack, chap and flake – something that saliva makes worse – usually when it's cold. So when the temperature drops make sure you have got a decent balm to seal them against the weather. If they are already chapped, use an old toothbrush or flannel to exfoliate them gently (lip *exfoliators*? What a waste of money!), and keep them coated with balm day and night for a few days.

'don't put lip balm on immediately before lipstick as it will fade the colour faster. Give balm time to absorb and plump-up lips, then blot with a tissue to take off any extra greasiness if you need to'

shopping for lip treatments

Before you head for the shops or flash your cash:

1. Find out whether the lip balm has a protective filter in it – your lips need first-line UV defence – unless you plan to wear protective lipstick.
2. Decide whether you are buying the lip balm or the pot – some balms come in swanky pots and tubes that are designed to look good when you get them out of your handbag, and it's easy to be swayed by the packaging.
3. Decide how much you want to spend: it was a question of extremes with our testers – they liked the real cheapies or seriously spenny ones.

... lipcare products we rate:

Julia Elizabeth Arden Eight Hour Cream (£13 for 50ml): 'I've used Eight Hour Cream since I was a little Pony Clubbing girl and I'm afraid nothing else comes close.'

Kate Gatineau Electelle Beautifying Lip Care (£17.75 for 15ml): 'I've got a tube of this in my car, on my desk and in the pocket of my dog-walking coat. It's a lip cream not a balm and I like to smother loads and loads of it on.'

the top 5 lip care products

the mission: To find you the most effective and user-friendly lip care products on the market.

the criteria Our testers judged the lip care products they tried on their ability to relieve dryness and chapping primarily, but also to make lips smoother and more plump (although most of our testers were realistic about this and did not expect to see a significant difference in lip volume). They also judged the products on how long they lasted (those that felt too slippery or migrated downwards were dismissed) and the key features – their taste and smell.

Vaseline Lip Therapy Petroleum Jelly

99p for 20gm

Although a few of you don't like the taste of this, most of you agreed that this is the best value lip emollient on the market. 'You can't fault its moisturising properties,' says Katie (21), 'it's my little saviour.' Doreen (56) doesn't wear lipstick because she can't bear the taste of it, but is 'very happy' to wear this. 'It's the only thing I like on my lips other than food!' she says.

the science bit: There isn't much of a secret to this formula – it is based on the super lubricant petroleum jelly.

Kiehl's Lip Balm SPF15

£6.50 for 15ml

We didn't realise how popular this balm was until we got our questionnaires back and saw all your positive comments on it. One tester, Karen (33) said, 'Someone bought me some in America once and I've never been out of it since. It's good because it's the only balm I've tried that isn't too greasy or minty – I hate the way some of them feel like they've set your lips on fire – and it keeps your lips nice and supple.' Another tester, Annette (47), who spends lots of time outdoors with her horses said, 'I've never bothered with lip balm in my life – it's all new to me, but this has been a real saviour for me over the past few months. Thanks.'

the science bit: The emollient formula contains sweet almond and wheat-germ oils, moisturising aloe vera and squalene, a softening ingredient.

Crème De La Mer Lip Balm

£35 for 9gm

We had a bet as to how this balm would go down with our testers. We thought they would say it was no better than any other and the expense was just marketing hype. But none of them did: Cathy (58) and Lottie (35) both asked to try it because they had read so much about the cream, and absolutely loved it. 'It's the smoothest, creamiest balm I've ever used. It just feels incredibly expensive, you can tell it's got really good ingredients in it,' said Cathy. 'The minty flavour is just right,' said Lottie, 'not too strong or lingering. And it makes your lips feel like velvet. I'd buy it.'

the science bit: The formula contains the so-called 'miracle broth' that is also in the cream, but applied to the balm via a distillation process, and in much higher concentration. It has also got a special Arctic marine anti-freeze protein in it.

Elizabeth Arden Eight Hour Cream Lip Protectant Stick

£13 for 3.7gm

'I love this. I always used Eight Hour Cream on my lips as balm anyway without realising you could get it as an actual balm!' said Paula (24), one of three people who gave this product full marks. 'It's very soothing, it doesn't melt and smudge which a lot of lip balms do, and it smells divine. It's a lot of money for a lip balm but I'd probably pay it.' Genevieve (35) said 'it's the WD40 of the beauty world.'

the science bit: The key ingredients are petrolatum – a skin lubricant and protectant – antioxidant vitamin E, salicylic acid which has a healing and smoothing benefit, and a broadspectrum (UVA and UVB) filter (padimate O and oxybenzone).

Blistex Herbal Balm £2.25 for 4.25gm

'Not much I can say about this,' wrote Emily (31), 'except that it does what you want a lip balm to do – moisturises your lips and stops them from chapping. So it meets the criteria. It's a beauty classic, isn't it? It's also a good price, so you can rattle through it and buy two more to keep you going.'

the science bit: The balm contains soothing aloe vera and camomile extract, and the emollients shea butter and avocado oil.

eye treatments

The skin around your eyes is generally the first bit of your body to show the world how old you are – and, frustratingly, the hardest part to treat. There are various reasons for this. First, the skin is thinnest here than anywhere else on your body (even your chest and the backs of your hands); we're talking about 0.5mm thick (so wafer thin) as opposed to an average of 2.5mm on the rest of you. This is the main reason it ages so fast, but not the only one. Because your eyes are always moving, the skin is subjected to constant wear and tear. And if it's really unlucky it gets yanked around when you take off your make-up everyday as well. The upshot is lines and crow's feet – real signs of age. But the skin around your eyes can also get puffy and dark (underneath and in the corners), and although neither of these problems are necessarily caused by age they can be made worse by it.

'are the rumours true about certain brands of haemorrhoid cream being excellent at reducing dark circles? We can't *possibly* comment'

Naturally there is an army of eye gels, creams and emulsions to 'combat' these problems. But because the skin is so fine these should only ever be applied very gently and sparingly via fingertip, and not directly around your eyes. Knowing where to put eye cream and how much to apply is something that baffles a lot of you judging by your comments on our survey. Many of you also wondered out loud how long you have to use a product before it shifts dark circles or bags. Which speaks volumes about your understanding of eye-care products.

So how do you care for eye-zone skin? And what can you do to stop it from prematurely ageing? *Anything*? Yes. But first, get out your kid gloves ...

always

- Aim to keep friction and pulling to a minimum – whether cleansing or applying make-up to your eyes.
- Keep the skin around your eyes as supple as possible – dry skin ages faster. Oily cleansers help with this: even when you have removed them they normally leave your skin feeling supple, not taut.
- Use hypo-allergenic unfragranced products as far as possible: eyes are very sensitive and will react by puffing-up or stinging if they don't like a product – something that often happens when you apply sun-screens with chemical filters too close to your eyes.

never

- Sleep in your make-up: yes, we know 'slept-in mascara' can look surprisingly good the next morning, but this is a cardinal sin because make-up can dry out your skin and in this area it needs all the help it can get.
- Rub your eyes: constantly stretching the skin puts it under pressure and it won't always ping back so fast ...
- Smoke: it's up there with the sun as a *big* skin ager. Cigarette smoke contains millions of molecules called free radicals which age your skin when they come into contact with it. It also makes your skin grey because it literally smokes it (like salmon), and every time you drag on a cigarette and screw up your eyes elasticity breaks down and skin becomes less supple. You have been warned.

how to cleanse your eyes

1. Use a silicone or oil-based eye make-up remover or ordinary cleanser (as long as it's safe to use in this area) and lots of it.
2. There are a few ways to cleanse your eyes: we think the best way is to apply make-up remover or cleanser by hand, massaging it into the skin around and over your eyes very gently with a fingertip, and then removing it – and the make-up – by pressing a damp flannel against your eyes, rinsing and applying it again until all the make-up has gone. This technique works best with oily make-up removers or water-soluble cleansers. If you use wipe-off cleanser or make-up remover, saturate a cottonwool bud and use it the same way, dabbing it onto your eyes, holding it there for a few seconds, then removing and doing it again. Whatever you do though, *don't wipe* your skin. Pat your skin dry with a towel.

popular eye problems sorted

- **dark under-eye circles** are as misunderstood as cellulite – which is saying something! So what are they? Blood vessels, usually. Because the skin here is so thin and transparent, you can see the underlying blood vessels through it. It's as simple as that, although sometimes – in the case of darker skins – the darkness can be pigmentation. When people say they have 'bags' under their eyes because they are tired what they usually mean is that the dark circles look worse, which is quite possible. So can you erase them? Not completely, no. Some people say eye creams help, so can be worth investigating ones which aim to reduce dark circles. But we swear by water – drinking enough of it eases blocked lymph and a sluggish system and makes the area look clearer – together with a concealer which has lots of pigment in it (so a little goes a long way) and doesn't dry on your skin. Concealers are especially useful if the dark circles are a pigmentation problem. Find out which ones are worth buying in the section on make-up (see page 135).
- **puffiness** – there are two types: the first is an all-over puffiness which we usually experience after a late night, wearing too heavy cream on our eyes, as an allergic reaction or at the wrong time of the month when fluid retention kicks in. Again, some people swear by cooling eye gels, saying they help to take puffiness down. But if it's something that happens a lot you could try eating less salt and processed foods, and drinking more water to flush out excess trapped fluid. The other type is the puffy under-eye 'bags', which usually appear with age as the fat pads that cushion your eyes begin to pull away from the bone of the lower eye and sag. If this is your problem you can only be clever with your eye make-up: aim for soft definition with muted colours – so brown mascara instead of black and neutral eyeshadows with a satin finish. Keep the underside of your eyebrows tidy and wear pearlised highlighting shadow on your brow bones – both help to 'open up' the eye area and 'lift' droopy eyes.

which eye care product do you need?

- Gel – can moisturise but also has a cooling effect on your skin. It may contain ingredients that help drain excess fluid from the tissues near your eyes, so helping to take down puffiness.
- Cream – can be the most moisturising, but it is *not necessarily any lighter in texture than an ordinary face cream.* Can contain draining ingredients and light-reflective particles to help make fine lines in the area look less obvious by bouncing light off them in a flattering way.
- Emulsion – halfway between a cream and a gel, it feels light and cool but still creamy, and can also contain drainage ingredients, light-reflectors or be pearlised.

shopping for eye care products

Before you head for the shops or flash your cash:

1. Decide whether you really need an eye care treatment or whether you can deal with a problem like dark under-eye circles or puffiness another way (like drinking more water and not covering your eyes with heavy creams at night).
2. Check to see if the product is scented – we would not recommend using highly fragranced products in this sensitive area.
3. Be realistic about the benefits you want and the claims made by the product. If an eye cream's *sole claim* is to 'erase' dark under-eye circles (rather than 'soften' or 'reduce' them – which it may be able to do if it contains light-reflectors or ingredients that drain excess fluid from the tissues) don't buy it. You will be wasting your money – as one of our testers, Vicki (40), discovered. She told us that she has 'spent a fortune on under-eye creams to remove dark circles and none of them has worked'. Think about it: how can a topical product 'erase' blood vessels under your skin? Exactly. On the other hand, if a product makes claims to erase them but says it will *also* moisturise and you like the way it feels and smells, you could use your discretion and perhaps overlook its wilder claims.
4. Decide how much you want to spend: our road tests proved that you can buy really good eye care products from both ends of the market – cheap and premium.

... eye care treatments we rate:

Julia Estée Lauder Advanced Night Repair Eye Recovery Complex (£29 for 15ml): 'I must admit that eye creams have never really appealed to me. I used to feel that creams just sat there making my eyes look baggier while gels are more cooling – they give your eyes a little wake-up call. This treatment is unique in that it's refreshing and light, yet it's also a cream. I was impressed by its performance too – I swear it made a difference to my dark circles.'

Kate Clarins Instant Eye Make-Up Remover (£12 for 125ml): 'I'm a bit lazy about eye creams, but I do use a special remover to take off mascara because I'm fantatical about not pulling the skin. And I'll definitely be road-testing Clarins Beauty Flash for Eyes when it finally appears.'

the 6 best eye treatments

the mission To find you the most effective and user-friendly eye care treatments on the market.

the criteria Our testers judged the eye care products they tried for their ability to hydrate, firm and refresh the skin around their eyes, as well as their ability to 'soften' fine lines and dark under-eye circles, and reduce puffiness.

Estée Lauder Lightsource Age-Resisting Eye Cream

£27 for 15ml

Jaqi (65) thought this eye cream was excellent. She said, 'It's cool and refreshing and surprisingly it didn't make my eyes puffy as have eye creams I've used in the past.' Another tester, Dawn (59) was amazed by the way it made the lines around her eyes look less noticeable: 'I've never had success with an eye cream like this,' she noted, asking 'What's the magic ingredient because whatever it is, it works!'

the science bit: The formula contains antioxidant vitamins E and C, which help to neutralise the ageing effects of free radicals on the skin – so slowing down ageing – plus algae and yeast to retain moisture. But the really clever features are light-reflectors which ping light away from lines making them less obvious.

Amirose Revitalising Cucumber Eye Pads

£2.29 for 10 pads

Why bother buying cucumber look-a-like cotton pads for your eyes when you could just slice up the real thing for free? Our thoughts entirely. But the people who tried these pads tell us we are wrong because they loved them, saying they sit nicely over the eye socket and have a pleasant moisturising effect. Emily (31) says, 'They worked well against my expectations, giving me eyes that feel and look fresher and clearer.' Like us, Molly (27) thought they would be a waste of money until she tried them and then asked Julia if she could have another pack. Cheeky.

the science bit: The pads are packed with soothing, cooling, diuretic ingredients – camomile, cucumber, aloe vera, green tea (an antioxidant).

Molton Brown Eye Rescue

£22 for 15ml

A cooling emulsion which Anna (24) loves because 'the cooling effect it has around my eyes also makes the skin there feel tighter. The lines haven't done a disappearing act though'. Jo (38) was impressed by the lightness of this cream and says it manages to 'slightly lift and soften the darkness near my eyes which means I don't have to be so heavyhanded with concealer'.

the science bit: Contains liposomes which carry its active ingredients – including starflower oil, which causes that tightening sensation – into the skin.

Farmacia Spa Therapy Eye Compress & Lotion Kit

£25 for 2 month's supply

'These are wonderfully refreshing, but you need to use them while lying down otherwise you get jelly-like worms sliding down your face,' said Joan (45). Not the quickest treatment in the book – you need about 15 minutes to lie back with them – and a couple of our testers wondered who would have the time for this. But everyone agreed that the results are impressive: 'You get instantly fresher and wide awake eyes,' said Joan. 'And it's marvellous at taking down puffiness.'

the science bit: The kit includes eye compresses (five packs of them) that you spray with the eye lotion, then place under your eyes for ten to 15 minutes.

Talika Eye Therapy Patch

£28 for 6 pairs of patches (each patch is re-usable up to four times).

Not an everyday treatment – you need a good spare 20 to 30 minutes to get a genuine reduction in puffiness, but if you can spare the time our testers think you won't regret it. 'I've had a professional Talika eye treatment, which I loved,' wrote Anna (42), 'and they used this product in the treatment, so I was really pleased to be able to use it at home. It's a good excuse to lie down with your feet up for a while, too.'

the science bit: The patches contain a blend of good quality essential oils with diuretic benefits, ceramides and karate, a nourishing skin nutrient.

Superdrug Vitamin E Contour Eye Gel

£1.99 for 15ml

The bargain of the bunch – our testers loved it, despite its rather basic packaging and simple formula. Nancy (47) said, 'It's a light, non-sticky gel and you dot it around your eyes – cooling, nourishing and for very little money.'

the science bit: The main ingredient is vitamin E, reparative, antioxidant and nourishing – simple, but clearly effective.

skin primers

Skin primers are a fairly new invention (you see them in lots of the contemporary expert make-up lines) and, as far as we're concerned, they have become an entirely necessary one! So what are they? Well, the basic idea is that they help to maximise the appearance of your skin whether or not you decide to wear make-up on top. Some primers aim to make your skin matt so that foundation (and other make-up) goes on easier and stays on for longer; others have a hint of iridescence or pearlescence in them which helps to improve the look of your skin by reflecting light off it in a flattering way.

So who needs them? Anyone who finds that their make-up does a disappearing act halfway through the day or thinks their skin needs a little extra help to look great. And whose doesn't?

what makes a good primer?

Primers come in various forms, and like many beauty products the best ones do *one* job well. These are the main benefits:

- Temporarily firming skin – primers with a gel-like or egg-like consistency can make skin look more toned and feel smoother.
- Highlighting strategic areas – primers with a hint of iridescence, apricot or metallic tint can be dotted onto upper cheekbones and forehead and make your complexion look healthier and more vital.
- Softening lines and blemishes – primers with light-reflective pigments can conceal or play down lines and blemishes by deflecting light away from them.
- Making make-up more durable – primers with mattifying properties (like powder) can help to make foundation and blusher cling harder to your skin, so enhance your make-up's staying-power.

when do you need primer?

1. When you want your make-up to stay in place without needing to be retouched until you take it off at night.
2. When your skin needs a little pick-me-up after a late night or a few too many drinks.
3. When you don't want full foundation coverage but still need to put fine lines into 'soft focus'.
4. When your skin is tanned and you want to enhance it and make it sparkle.
5. When you want the sheerest face base possible – just touches of it to highlight your face.

‘pearlescent or iridescent skin primers can be used as face highlighters – in other words, you just 'touch' them onto strategic points like your temples, brow and cheekbones instead of applying a light veil of primer all over your face’

is it worth spending money on eye & lip primers or 'bases'?

Probably not. It is tricky to get make-up to stay put around your eyes and on your lips. But there are better (and cheaper) ways to stop colour pigment from falling into your eyelid creases or leaking into the fine lines around your mouth. Most eye shadow primers are very similar to cream-to-powder eye shadow and foundation formulas.

shopping for skin primers

Before you head for the shops or flash your cash:

1. Decide what kind of skin primer you want – one that creates a matt base for your skin and helps to keep your make-up on, or one that makes your skin more radiant – there are lots of choices.
2. If you are buying a light-reflective primer make sure it's a good quality one with very fine mirrored particles in it.
3. Decide how much you want to spend: most of the primers that came out well in our road tests were from the more expensive end of the market, although Face Lift – a primer developed by top make-up artist Barbara Daly and very competitively priced – was among those rated the best.

'to perk up tired skin, mix a tiny bit of iridescent primer with your daytime moisturiser and apply the two together (this works very well over a tan, too)'

... skin primers we rate:

Julia La Prairie Cellular Rose Illusion Line Filler (£65 for 30ml): 'It's like putting on a new skin and fantastic as a base for foundation. Worth every single penny!'

Kate Guerlain Divinora Pure Radiance (£35 for 30ml): 'An all-time fave of mine – I first discovered it when I was working on a magazine nearly two decades ago and I've never been without a bottle of it since. I usually wear it on its own over moisturiser. It's a clear gel with 9-carat gold flakes suspended in it which melt when you apply it, and if you put it on just after cleansing and moisturising it traps the warmth in and makes your skin look toned and pink.'

the 7 best skin primers

the mission To find you the most effective and user-friendly skin primers on the market.

the criteria Our testers judged the face primers they tried on their ability to enhance the skin – either by making it appear less lined, brighter and more radiant, healthier-looking, firmer, more lifted, more matt or smooth. They also judged face primers on how well they assisted make-up application and stability.

Shiseido The Make-Up Smoothing Veil SPF15 £22 for 50ml

A base which can be used on its own or under make-up and aims to make skin a flawless canvas – blurring fine lines and creating a translucent finish. Our tester, Joy (63), said she has 'no hesitation in recommending this product at all. It creates a good base for your make-up and it really improves its staying-power'. Louise (32) said, 'It's good for pale skins because it gives it a bit of much-needed radiance.'

the science bit: It incorporates Shiseido's Advanced Luminous Technology – a clever use of prismatic powders to balance skin colour (it brightens dull, dark skin very well) – and can be worn alone or under foundation or powder.

Bio-Col Velvet Skin £52 for 15ml

'I'm at an age where my face is beyond repair so it was nice to use something that really did make a difference to my skin and my make-up. I truly did look better for it,' said Lou (68). Another tester, Frances (42) said she thought 'it was good value because a tiny drop of it goes a long way; it must have some very clever ingredients in it to make it go over your skin so smoothly. It's as if it's on wheels'.

the science bit: As well as mattifying and smoothing skin ready for make-up, this primer treats your skin – its main active ingredient is retinyl palmitate, a derivative of vitamin A, which has proved to increase production of collagen and elastin.

Laura Mercier Foundation Primer £26 for 50ml

French make-up artist Laura Mercier was one of the pioneers of make-up primers and this one – developed by her – is still one of the best. 'It's hard to describe,' wrote Katie (39), 'but the best way to describe its effects is to say that it seems to keep my face in place.' Sophie (40) tried it without foundation: 'I don't wear foundation much but I need more than moisturiser and I thought this would fill the gap. It did – it made my skin look smooth and slightly sheeny – but I still needed a bit of blusher.'

the science bit: A blend of lavender, orange, rose, jasmine, honey, green tea and geranium extracts, and Laura Mercier recommends gently massaging the primer into your skin until it loses its 'wet feel' to stimulate skin and circulation.

Clarins Beauty Flash Balm £21.50 for 50ml

We have yet to find someone who doesn't rate this product – and a few of our testers actually asked us if they could road test it for us because they had read so much about it. 'A miracle in a tube,' said Jane (40). 'Can't live without it,' wrote Georgie (55). Industry insiders – make-up artists and beauty editors – call it 'Cinderella in a tube' because it is such a great instant fix for skin that needs perking up. One tip: use it sparingly, otherwise it peels off when you apply foundation over the top.

the science bit: The emulsion has a consistency like egg white, so sets skin with a firming film; it is also slightly iridescent, so helps to play down fine lines and give skin a flattering glow.

Revlon Skinlights Face Illuminator £9.95 for 40ml

Best for bare skin, enhancing a tan – and for beginners: 'I've never even heard of skin primers,' wrote Annie (26), 'so it was a relief to be given this to test because it's so easy to use. I just dotted it onto my cheeks and forehead and rubbed it in. I was amazed at how it 'picked up' my skin; I definitely look healthier with it on.'

the science bit: This is a primer and highlighting fluid with rose quartz, mother-of-pearl or topaz iridescent particles which can be used on its own and applied to strategic areas (cheek and brow bones, temples), mixed with moisturiser, or used to prime skin before foundation.

Face Lift By Barbara Daly For Tesco £6 for 30ml

This was discontinued and then brought back by popular demand – the testers who liked it (and women we spoke to who have tried it before) all said it is a miracle in a bottle and a supermarket bargain. 'I can't be doing with all the fancy brands,' said Caroline (42). 'I buy most of my beauty products in the supermarket, and I was so chuffed to discover this. It's really helpful – especially on days when your skin needs a bit of extra help (most days for me). The thing I like most about it is the fact that it firms and lifts your skin subtly – so you don't get that unnaturally tight look around your eyes – and your skin feels comfortable underneath, not horrible and tight.'

the science bit: The formula includes collagen-strengthening vitamin E, anti-oxidant vitamin E, and an SPF of 10.

DDF Wrinkle Relax (originally known as Faux-Tox) £75 for 15ml

This stuff got acres of editorial coverage when it was first launched – for a reason: 'It's a total life-saver,' wrote Vicky (40). 'I bought some after reading about it in one of the glossy mags and couldn't believe it. When people say it's like botox without the needles they're right – I don't know why anyone would spend money on those injections when they can get the same effect from a bottle – but I think it does even more for you than that. You put it on under your foundation and you just look more rested, which does wonders for the way your skin looks.' And that sort of says it all really.

the science bit: The key ingredient is a hexa peptide – one of the most advanced ingredients currently being used in skin care – which stimulates the muscle, and this ultimately has a tightening and firming effect on skin.

skin problem solvers

Spots – what are they then? Only joking! We all get them – always, always when (and where) we least want them – i.e., before a big date or important interview.

Beauty writers are not immune either: because our lives are one long beauty road test we can suffer from problems like spots, rashes and dry patches on a regular basis. Kate started a new job editing the beauty pages of a magazine a few years ago with only half her face – the other half had peeled off over the previous weekend while she was trying out a 'miraculous' new face cream. Try living that down.

'never pick or squeeze spots – however tempting it might be – you will always regret it the next day, if not sooner'

The responses to our survey showed that most of you know that genes are the main factor behind the skin you have and – to a large extent – the way it behaves. But understandably you still want quick superficial antedotes to problems like spots, 'morning-after' skin, hyper-pigmentation and under-eye circles. (A couple of testers wanted an express self-tan remover, but we can't help you on that one yet – sorry).

Several of the people who answered our questionnaires wanted to know why beauty companies 'keep bringing out new "solutions" which claim to be even more of an amazing breakthrough but are often no better and sometimes completely useless?'. Er, how long have you got? No, seriously, the short answer to this is that beauty is like any other business (its main aim is to make money), but most of the houses are also genuinely dedicated to bringing us the latest, most effective skin care solutions. Promise.

The best way forward with skin problems is first to identify what sort of snags you run up against most – be it blackheads, dry patches or whatever – so you know which troubleshooters you need on emergency standby in your bathroom cabinet. Then all you need to know is which ones are worth buying. Which is where this book and our intrepid testers come in:

dry, flaky patches These can be caused by sleeping in your make-up, drying skin products and even too-heavy moisturisers which cause blocked pores and a build-up of dead skin cells.

- **myth**: that dry, flaky patches can be cured by expensive 'super' balms which claim to give intensive hydration.
- **answer**: lightweight moisturising creams and a consistent skincare regime.

brown/liver/sun/age spots (melasma) This occurs when melanin collects in one area of the skin. It can be caused by sun exposure, enlarged freckles, birth control pills, pregnancy or oestrogen replacement therapy.

- **myth**: that these spots are caused by liver problems; despite the name they are sometimes given they have nothing to do with your liver.
- **answer**: skin 'lightening' products – if the pigment is superficial and only as deep as the epidermis (most are). These are often a mix of ingredients like alpha hydroxy acids (AHAs) and hydroquinone or kojic acid – a by-product in the fermentation of saké, the Japanese rice wine.

NB For information on covering pigmentation problems like port wine stains go to the foundation and concealer chapters in the section on make-up (see pages 126 and 135).

spots These can be caused by hormones, overproduction of oil by oil glands, a build-up of bacteria inside pores, irregular shedding of dead skin cells on the surface of your skin and inside its pores. Teenagers are not the only sufferers either; many older people get spots and need a good remedy – of which lots of the people who took part in our survey reminded us.

- myth: that spots can be 'drawn' or 'dried' out; that they are caused by eating chips and chocolate, or that they can be instantly zapped into oblivion.
- answer: antiseptic treatments, medicated cleansers and non-comedogenic (non-pore clogging) moisturisers. If spots persist, consult your GP.

enlarged pores Nothing makes pores bigger except the natural ageing process; you either have small or large pores.

- myth: that pores can be 'closed' or 'minimised' by topical beauty products – especially astringent toner – or cold water; lots of our testers asked whether this is possible. Your skin might feel temporarily tighter, but the answer is no.
- answer: light-reflective skin primer, foundation or concealer. See the skin primer and make-up sections (see pages 48 and 125) for our testers' verdicts on which ones work best.

red rash or high colour This can occur as an allergic reaction to an ingredient or if your skin is hypersensitive and reacts with temperature changes, sun exposure and even after eating spicy food or drinking alcohol.

- myth: that this always automatically means you have got sensitive skin.
- answer: unscented, hypo-allergenic or dermatologic-tested soothing products. If the problem persists, consult your GP.

rosacea A nightmare (and very common) problem which develops over time as red and often dry skin with some acne features and in a 'butterfly' pattern over cheeks, but no one is exactly sure why, which makes it difficult to treat.

- myth: that it only affects pale, Caucasian skins.
- answer: very gentle skincare products, consultation with a dermatologist (you can usually get a referral from your GP) who may prescribe antibiotics and topical treatments. Avoid anything with retin-A, alpha or beta hydroxy acids (AHAs and BHAs), scent, menthol, peppermint, witch hazel, alcohol or eucalyptus in it as these ingredients can make rosacea flare up.

> 'if you have oily skin and use powder to mattify the surface be sure to cleanse thoroughly everyday because you can find that a build-up of powder can clog pores leading to an outbreak of spots or dry patches'

shopping for problem solvers

Before you head for the shops or flash your cash:

1. Decide whether you really need a problem solver or a regime revamp: are you getting spots or redness because your skin doesn't like the products you are using (they may be too harsh or not thorough enough), and are you being realistic about what you can 'solve' (i.e. closing 'open' pores)?
2. Check the ingredients – some might solve one problem but create another. For example, alpha hydroxy acids (AHAs) can make dry skin smoother but make rosacea worse.

... problem-solvers we rate:

Julia Origins Spot Remover (£8.50 for 10ml): 'You can't beat it. It stings like mad but it can kill spots off overnight.'

Kate 'My biggest skin problem is psoriasis which I get in patches on different bits of my body, and the only over-the-counter remedy is aqueous cream which you can buy in big tubs very cheaply from most chemists.'

the 7 best skin problem solvers

the mission To find you the most effective and user-friendly problem solvers on the market.

the criteria Our testers judged the problem solvers they tried on their ability to make a marked difference to the problem they were treating, be it spots or blocked pores, depressed-looking skin, high colour – even rosacea. They also judged the products they tried on their efficacy and instructions.

Bioré Deep Cleansing Nose Strips £7.50 for 6 strips

OK we admit it – we are addicted to these brilliant pore 'plasters'; there is something incredibly satisfying about ripping them off your nose and looking at what you have removed with them. We are not the only ones; all the people who tried them for us (or had used them previously), agreed that they are the best you can buy. 'There are imitations,' said Sally (26), 'and I've tried them all, but I still think these do the job best. They're quick, easy and seem to get out the most grime.'

the science bit: A magic ingredient called C-bond is the secret to the effectiveness of these strips; it locks onto the dirt in your pores and on your skin's surface.

Elemis SOS Emergency Cream

£26 for 30ml

This little wonder is renowned for being a really effective troubleshooter for a range of skin problems from sensitivity and high colour to sun-burn. 'I thought this cream made such a difference to my face I even put it on my shoulders where I'd had too much sun to soothe and repair the damage,' says Catherine (40), one of the testers who tried this product for us. 'It's incredibly soothing – I think it really comes into its own when you've had a bit too much sun – and it smells divine. I've finished it – can you get me some more?'

the science bit: The key ingredients are lavender and centella asiatica – both dynamic skin healers – soothing rice starch, meadowsweet (a natural anti-inflammatory so it can stop itching), and regenerative myrrh essential oil.

Gatineau Anti-Redness Cream

£30 for 50ml

'I have a classic English Rose complexion, and I find whenever I go into a pub my cheeks go bright red and stay that way all evening,' said Tessa (35). We gave her this product to try and she gave it 10/10 because she said it met the criteria and worked better – and faster – than any treatment she has tried so far. 'I felt much less of a burn on my face and I didn't look as flushed, so something was definitely working,' she said.

the science bit: The product improves the skin's micro-circulation, which helps excess blood near the skin's surface to flow back into the system; it also contains light-reflectors which soften existing redness, sunscreens to protect against further redness and comforting sweet almond and silk extracts.

Australian Bodycare Tea Tree Oil

£3.99 for 15ml

There appears to be nothing this little miracle can't do, so it's hardly surprising that when we asked people if they would like to try it out for us – on spots, athlete's foot or any other problem – they said they didn't need to because they already had it in the bathroom cabinet. 'I'm never out of it – but then it does take a long time to use up,' said Susie (31). 'I travel a lot and I always take it with me because it works so well on everything, taking the redness out of spots and bites. It even soothes sunburn.'

the science bit: A natural antiseptic, tea tree oil was used by the Aborigines in medicine and is used more and more by orthodox doctors to treat skin disorders.

DDF Rosacea Relief

£48 for 1oz

DDF stands for Doctor's Dermatologic Formula, a range developed by Dr Howard Sobel to treat skin problems. This is one of the heroes: 'I'm naturally sceptical about products that claim to help rosacea, especially if they're not medical, because I've had it for many years and have only ever come across a few treatments that made any difference,' said Rosemary (56). 'But I have to say this is one of them. I won't say my rosacea has gone, but it's not so angry – or dry for that matter. I'll keep using it.'

the science bit: The key agent is Gatuline A, and its main benefit is reducing inflammation; it also contains yeast extract, said to enhance healing, cocoa extract to increase circulation and lemon extract to clarify skin.

Dermalogica Skin Brightening System

£68 for the 3-product system

A skin care system that aims to even up skin tone and texture: 'I have to say it made a big difference to my skin; it looks much fresher and brighter,' said Anna (24). 'I found the regime a bit involved and tedious, but it has definitely changed the way my skin looks.' Julia is a big fan of this treatment, too; she thought it made a significant different to the pigmentation problems she had during her pregnancies.

the science bit: The regime involves applying Day Bright over moisturiser as a protective cover from ultraviolet (UV) light – it has a sun protection filter (SPF) of 15 – exfoliating with Daily Microfoliant in the evening and then applying Night Bright, a night-time serum.

Clinique Anti-Blemish Solutions Back & Chest Spray

£13 for 100ml

We think this is a really clever solution to an age-old problem: how do you treat a spotty back with medicated creams or washes unless you have got extraordinarily long arms? 'I get spots on my back quite a lot,' says Eve (37), 'I've been told it's to do with sweat and blocked pores and I usually just sit it out and wait for them to go. I thought it would be worth giving this spray a go – you never know when you're going to need it, and I found that it makes your skin feel less oily, so I assume this stops the oil collecting in the pores and forming spots. I've used it a few times on my back and have definitely had fewer spots.'

the science bit: Free of oil and fragrance, the spray works to clean pores and reduce the redness caused by spots.

SUN CARE

Sun care or sun *scare*?

Most of us now know that there is a downside to sunbathing. But what is the real story here? Is the sun a genuine threat to the health and youthfulness of your skin? Or is there just one big conspiracy going on to try and make us buy more sunscreens?

Well, you are reading the right book if you want to find out because if anyone is going to tell it to you straight, we are. The bare facts are that yes, the sun is *definitely* a threat to your health, and exposure to it – protected or not – ages your skin prematurely.

Put simply, UV exposure – and that means anything from lying by the pool to driving along in your car on a cloudy autumn day (UV rays are present all year round, not just in the summer) – can give you skin cancer and make your skin wrinkled, leathery, and uneven in tone quicker than it would if you covered up and blocked out the rays.

This is what is meant by the 'downside' of the sun.

On the upside, the sun – and exposure to it – makes us feel GOOD: more upbeat, happier and, when we get a bit of a tan, more confident, slimmer and healthier.

These positive feelings should not be underestimated: they are very significant – the reasons why we enjoy the sun and want a tan. The sun care companies know this. That is why they invest so much in developing sunscreens that help us get a tan 'safely'.

While there is no such thing as a safe tan, you can make the process as safe as possible by going about it sensibly. We will show you how – and reveal which are the best sunscreens and sun care products.

What you will find out about in this chapter:

- What kind of sunscreens are best for *your* skin
- The (significant) difference between mineral and chemical sunscreens
- Why some self-tans pong and others don't
- Why lying on a sunbed is quite possibly the worst beauty crime you can commit
- The difference between aftersun and normal body lotion

self-tan products

So who were those giant smelly carrots?

Us – and *you* – before self-tan became the marvellous impersonator it is today! It has also become seriously big business – hardly surprising when you think what a bad press sunbathing gets. The more we know about the perils of sun exposure the better self-tans get: the competition is on for sun care companies to make one which looks and feels as close and good to the real thing as possible. And they are doing very well.

> 'self-tanned skin isn't protected from the sun. And self-tans which have an SPF only give enough protection if you put them on just before or during sun exposure'

Mind you, things couldn't have got much worse. If you were brave enough to use the stuff a few years ago you ran the risk of turning orange; streaks and a strange telltale smell were not optional either. But judging by our testers' comments on their questionnaires, it appears that there is still some way to go: requests included 'a fake tan that lasts for at least a month before it needs topping up again' and 'something that removes self-tan streaks'. In both cases we reckon it is probably only a matter of time.

Despite the overall progress some self-tans haven't changed – they still do the same humiliating things to you. Others are so much better that they deserve a new name. Read on to find out which ones they are.

how to use self-tan

Don't skip this bit because you think you have read it a hundred times before: there is no point splashing out on a good self-tan if you don't put it on properly:

1. **Exfoliate everywhere** you intend to put self-tan – the point of doing this is to get rid of a build-up of dead skin on your body which makes self-tan look uneven and come off more quickly (when you lose the dead skin).
2. **Moisturise your whole body** – self-tan clings to moisturised skin better than dry.
3. **Apply self-tan in long sweeping movements** and swiftly without massaging it in too much.

4. **Wipe over heavily-lined areas** like your knees, heels and elbows with a flannel or damp cottonwool pad to stop self-tanning pigment from collecting in the lines.
5. **Allow self-tan at least an hour** (no matter how quickly it claims to develop on the bottle) to absorb or develop before getting dressed or into bed.
6. **Reapply self-tan** as you need to (usually every three to four days) after exfoliating and moisturising again.

how does self-tan work?

It is very simple: all self-tans use the same ingredient – dihydroxyacetone (DHA) – to chemically turn your skin brown. DHA browns skin through its interaction with the amino acid arginine found in surface skin cells. Some self-tans contain more DHA than others; and the more a product contains, the faster self-tan browns your skin. DHA is what gives self-tan that – er – *distinctive* smell. But some companies have found better ways of masking this than others. Find out which in the results of our road test.

do tanning pills work?

It depends which ones you take and what you classify as a tan. There are two types of tanning pill (also called pre-tan accelerators): those that contain an ingredient called tyrosine that is needed by your body to produce melanin (which is what tans your skin). But, no matter how much tyrosine you take orally you won't tan unless your skin is exposed to UV rays. In other words, tyrosine-based pre-sun tanning pills are a waste of money. Other tanning pills contain beta carotene, the property that makes carrots orange and if you take enough of it (or eat enough carrots), it changes the colour of your skin. *To orange*. If this is the colour you want to be, fine. But our advice would be to give them both a miss and get yourself a decent self-tan.

temporary tans

No matter how good self-tanning formulas have got, lots of our testers said they still didn't want to use them – mostly for fear of turning themselves orange. Bronzing powders make good substitutes if you still want to give your face a bit of healthy colour. Sweep them over completely dry skin (i.e. with all traces of moisturiser absorbed) with a big, fat, soft brush to give skin an instant pick-me-up:

beauty scoop highly commends:

- Pupa Bronzing Powder (£12 for 11ml): 'just the right amount of sparkle', said Helena (15), 'very easy to put on – you just whisk it all over your face and chest with a brush. And the silvery packaging is supremely cool'.
- Lancôme Star Bronzer Compact Bronzing Powder for Face & Body SPF8 (£25 for 50ml): gives skin a sun-kissed look and is foolproof – you can't overdo it no matter how hard you try. Comes in 2 shades so works on all skin tones: Nourdjan (37) said it gave her Asian skin 'a beautiful discreet gold shimmer that didn't disappear'.

shopping for self-tans

Before you head for the shops or flash your cash:

1. Decide where you are going to use self-tan: some people (ourselves included) only use it on their legs and faces, others put it all over, and you can buy different formulations for your face and body.
2. Decide how much you want to spend: our testers found that you can find effective conventional self-tans in each of the different price brackets from competitive to premium, but that you need to pay a bit more for a good wash-off (temporary) face tint.

... self-tans we rate:

Julia Lancôme Flash Bronzer Instant Self-Tanning Body Spritz (£17 for 150ml): 'I only use self-tan on my face and legs – and even then only occasionally. I can't fault this product. It's so easy to use and you don't have to pfaff around waiting too long for it to dry.'

Kate Clarins Radiance & Self Tanning Cream Gel (£21.50 for 50ml): 'I'm a face and legs only girl for self-tan. I wear this on my face from May to September; I just top it up. It's idiot-proof – it still works even when you put it on in a hurry.'

the best fake tans

the mission to find you the most effective and user-friendly self-tans on the market.

the criteria our testers judged the self-tanners they tried on their ability to give skin the most realistic fake tan, the speed which the colour developed and the smell – whether it was bearable or telltale (important, because most of our testers said they thought self-tans still smelt awful). They also judged self-tans and wash-off tints on their ability to moisturise skin, ease of application, and lifespan.

the best 6 self-tans

L'Oréal Sublime Bronze Self Tanning Gel

£9.99 for 150ml

Annalise (25) said this was 'one of the best self tans', and although Bridget (38) wasn't convinced by the smell, she felt it 'lasted better than any other I have tried, and I really loved the way it made my skin feel so soft'. As well as smell, lasting qualities were really important to our testers. Lily (41) commented: 'I used this on my arms first of all and it lasted for at least five days before looking a bit tired – even then only I noticed this. It faded gradually rather than in patches. I then did my face and legs and got the same results. Really great stuff'. Our testers agreed that the tan was very realistic, and that it was a joy to apply because it is tinted so you can see where you are putting it.

the science bit: as well as the active tanning ingredient, it includes AHAs, the chemical skin-smoothers which L'Oréal say helps to prevent streakiness.

Clarins Tinted Self Tanning Face Cream

£13.50 for 50ml

Eve (37) is very fussy about self-tan; she says she has never found one she is 100 percent convinced by, and even though she wasn't mad about the smell of this product she still gave it a high rating because 'it gave me a really good healthy-looking tan, and although I'm fussy about self-tan I was impressed and would definitely buy it despite its smell'. Vicki (40) doesn't really use self-tan on her fair skin but was convinced by this one, saying 'it was really good and a great natural colour – I didn't look at all orange as I feared I would'. The added bonuses with this self-tan is that it has an SPF15 and it is tinted so it gives your skin an instant glow and you can see where you are applying it.

the science bit: as well as DHA, it contains skin conditioning and tanning ingredients ayapana, birch bark and olive leaf extracts.

Sisley Self Tanning Gel

£40 for 75ml

This is available in two shade formulas – one for fair skin and two for dark – and can be used on your face and body. 'Really impressed with this,' wrote Anneka (28), who used the formula for pale skin. 'I only used it on my face and even though I'm not a pro when it comes to self-tan I managed to get it on without any streaks – although I think that's down to the performance of the product rather than me – and all the colour I needed in one application.' 'More of a cream than a gel,' wrote Cindy (50), 'but a cream with a really light texture – superb. It works quite fast – just over an hour to a tan, so I was able to use it in the morning before getting dressed. I was pleasantly surprised by its smell. How much did you say it was?' £40. 'Is that the going price for a good self-tan?'

the science bit: as well as DHA, it contains an ingredient called erythulose which helps to prolong the colour, plus sesame and corn oil to hydrate and smooth skin.

Helena Rubinstein Golden Beauty Sun Tan Express Crystal Self-Tanning Gel

£18 for 50ml

This facial self-tan has a light, non-sticky gel texture, which went down well with our testers – 'It doesn't feel like you are going to make a mistake with a gel somehow,' said Laura (29), 'it must be psychological' – and seemed to give the speediest results; our two testers found that it developed in under an hour, which is impressive. 'I've always used this brand for self-tanners,' wrote Lottie (39). 'The shade is perfect. I've got quite fair skin and it just makes it look a bit warmer, and I think the colour is more natural than most self-tans because it's so subtle. It looks so fake when it's too dark and it makes you look ridiculous. It's also got a really lovely sunshine holiday smell to it.'

the science bit: as well as tanning ingredients, it contains micro-reflectors to enhance the look of skin and even out its tone, and antioxidant vitamin E.

L'Oréal Sublime Bronze Multi-Position Anti-Streaking Self-Tanning Spray

£9.99 for 125ml

All the testers who tried this self-tan for us – or had used it in the past – said they thought it was brilliant, mainly because it allows you to reach the parts that most fake tans don't because it is a spray. 'I only use self-tan on my face and sometimes my legs, but never the rest of my body,' wrote Kate (42). 'This is partly because I can't get there without my husband's help, and even then I worry that it hasn't gone on evenly. This was a real test to see if I could apply it all-over myself. You do need a mirror – and you have to be a bit of a contortionist to see what you're doing, and you need to wear a shower cap if you've got long hair, but I have to say the effects were very, very even. I was amazed at myself. And the tan is a good, natural colour.'

the science bit: contains alpha hydroxy acids (AHAs) which exfoliate skin – the idea being that the smoother your skin the more even the tan.

St Tropez Whipped Bronze Self Tanning Mousse

£20 for 4oz

St Tropez revolutionised the self-tanning business when they introduced their salon tanning treatment – with its unique application system – a decade ago. No surprise then that St Tropez is now synonymous with serious celebrity fake baking. 'I've never had the salon treatment but have read so much about it,' wrote Tamsin (32). 'I probably could do with a bit more practise at applying it. But the effects were fantastic, you can understand what all the fuss is about, and it lasted incredibly well – for at least five or six days. I'd love to buy this product.' Other bonuses: it doesn't smell and dries in about a minute. Our tip: wear plastic gloves or scrub your hands well after application.

the science bit: the updated formula contains aloe leaf juice and alpha hydroxy acids (AHAs) to limit streakiness and make the colour deeper and longer-lasting.

the best 3 wash-off skin tints

Guerlain Teint Doré

£15 for 125ml

Every time Guerlain think about discontinuing this product there is an outcry – which is why it has been around since the Second World War. There is reason why: it is a simple water-resistant formula – a liquid tint – which works extremely well. Kerry (39) was a little hesitant at first about using it, she thought it looked as if it would stain her skin (and clothes) and she would not be able to get it off if she made a mistake. 'I wasn't sure how to apply it as it's very runny,' she said. 'But I followed the instructions and it was easy. Such a nice colour, it looked like I'd had a weekend in the south of France. I love it.' Our tip: the best way to apply this product is to soak a cottonwool ball with it and stroke it lightly over your face.

the science bit: in a class of its own, this skin tint feels like water and has a high pigment content, so gives skin some realistic colour even when used sparingly. Best applied on a cottonwool square and stroked lightly over your face.

Becca Translucent Bronzing Gel

£25 for 50ml

Our testers gave this a high rating for two main reasons: it blends incredibly well into skin and its pump dispenser is practical and easy to use. Emma (34) was new to this cult make-up brand, developed by Australian make-up artist Rebecca Morrice-Adams, but was one of the testers who gave it 10/10: 'The colour is very natural, first class,' she said. 'It's a bit off-putting initially because it's very dark, but it soon blends into your skin. I looked so healthy I didn't bother with any other make-up.' Our tip: the best way to apply it is to pat it onto your forehead, cheeks and chin and blend it in with quick, feathery strokes.

the science bit: a really creamy gel which smoothes over skin like silk but feels cool and gives very sheer, even results. Best applied by patting it onto your forehead, chin and cheeks and blending it in with quick, feathery strokes.

Sex Symbol Aerotan £15.45 for 150ml

A temporary tan in a spray-on can – how easy can it get? 'Bloody marvellous,' wrote Hannah (31). This tan did the rounds with our testers and although all were dubious about trying it, most could not believe how good it was. It literally provides spray-on colour and can be used to enhance an existing tan, and give pale skin an instant or deepen darker-toned skin. 'I really loved this product. It's fun, easy to use and it turned me a great colour. I used it on my face and body,' says Jackie (49). Our tip: the best way to apply this product is to put it into the palms of your hands first, then smooth it over your face.

the science bit: the original 'tan in a can', this self-tan projects a fine and even spray onto skin (it is best applied from the palms of your hands rather than directly onto your body); it gives skin a flattering sheen and has the best scent of all self-tans – yummy coconut!

sunscreens

Most of us now know that we need to squeeze sunscreens in our suitcases when we go on holiday somewhere hot, even if the reasons why may not be entirely clear.

We don't blame you if you are baffled by sunscreens – at times we are too. You almost need a degree in biochemistry to get to grips with sun protection fully and just when you think you have, the information changes as the experts come up with new theories over the way the sun affects us and the best way to defend ourselves from it.

'if you only take one piece of advice from this book we hope it's that you don't use sunbeds'

Some basic and key facts never change though: when skin is exposed to the sun without protection it doesn't just burn, it ages faster – *much* faster – and more importantly, it increases the risk of you developing skin cancer. This is why sunscreens (the products you take on holiday and the screens that are added to your moisturiser or foundation) should play such a pivotal role in our skincare regimes – and our lives.

In this chapter we will reveal which the best sunscreens are, and give you some logical information about how to protect yourself properly while still getting a bit of a tan.

to tan or not to tan?

Sunbathing is the most damaging thing you can do to your skin and in an ideal world none of us would do it. But we do. And we do it because apart from the fact that it's lovely being in the warm sun, having a tan makes us feel good – for some, getting a tan is what a holiday is all about. There is no getting away from this, and we think it's unrealistic to advise people to stay out of the sun forever and never allow their skin to tan. The only compromise is to aim for a light, sun-kissed tan rather than all-out (and a bit naff) bronze, and to stay out of the sun from 11am to 2pm, when it's at its strongest. Whatever you do though, remember that any exposure to the sun – be it for a light tan or grilling – ages your skin and increases your risk of developing skin cancer.

how the sun affects your skin

- It emits ultraviolet (UV) wavelengths, two of which cause the most trouble: UVA rays age it (think UV**A** = Ageing), and UVB rays which burn and brown it (think UV**B** = Burning & Browning). Each of these rays boosts the effect of the other; they are both present everyday (so not just when you go on holiday or in summer time) even when it's cloudy, and UVA – the main cause of skin cancer – goes through glass.
- It triggers melanin, skin's natural pigment, which comes up to the surface of your skin as a defensive reaction and is equal to sun protection factor (SPF) 2 in sunscreen. This is why *all* skins – no matter what colour – need sunscreen.
- It activates free radicals – the molecules in your skin which actively age it – within five minutes of exposure, which makes wrinkles form faster and damages collagen (the stuff that makes skin springy and elastic), giving you that old leathery look.

‘there is no such thing as a ‘safe’ tan: the tan you get on Brighton beach is as much of a threat to your skin as baking your skin for two weeks on a beach in Spain’

bad reactions

When your skin gets irritated in the sun it's either caused by the UV rays, your sunscreen or other beauty products you have used before going in the sun:

- **if you suffer from photodermatosis**: wear a sunscreen with a higher SPF and ideally one with a mineral, not chemical, filter. These tend to be sunscreens which contain the ingredients titanium dioxide and zinc dioxide.
- **if your skin gets itchy and red** it may be a bad reaction to the combination of sun, sea and scented products: take unscented, hypo-allergenic beauty products on holiday.
- **if your skin stings** (usually around your eyes) when you apply sunscreen it may not like a chemical filter: swap to a mineral one.

making sense of sunscreens

This is where we explain to you how sunscreens work – it's important, so don't skip it!

1. **How to get the right level of protection**: sunscreens contain filters – sun protection filters (SPFs) – which are coded by number and the higher the number, the longer the sunscreen allows you to be in the sun (or exposed to UVB rays – the ones that burn and brown your skin). The first thing you have to do is work out how long you can stay in the sun *without sunscreen on* before you start to go pink or burn. For both of us it's about 15 minutes. Once you have decided this, all you need to do is to multiply this time with the SPF number on your sunscreen. So if it's SPF30, you multiply 30 by 15 to get your answer – 450 minutes or 7½ hours.
2. **How to get the best quality protection**: your sunscreen must give you broad spectrum protection from UV rays. This means it protects you from both UVA *and* UVB rays – not just UVB, which is often the case. If you are not sure, check the ingredients (see Shopping for sunscreens on page 70) or ask for advice.

waterproof v water-resistant

Surprise, surprise – there is no such thing as a waterproof sunscreen: all sunscreens should be reapplied after you have been swimming or worked up a sweat in the sun. But water-resistant sunscreens are formulated to stay on longer than waterproof, so this could be the factor that sways you when you are looking for the best sunscreens.

how to sunbathe safely

- **pale skin** – has poor inbuilt defence: it's most prone to sun damage because it has the least amount of natural melanin.
  we recommend: 'non-chemical' sunscreens (with inert ingredients) that won't irritate sensitive pale skins.
- **dark skin** – has medium inbuilt defence: it has more melanin, but dark skin is no thicker than pale, burns and inflames easily and is prone to hyperpigmentation.
  we recommend: suncare products with anti-inflammatory agents like aloe vera.
- **olive skin** – has high inbuilt defence: it's got more pigment than pale skin but is more olive than brown in tone. So it has more natural protection than pale skin but less of an exaggerated hyperpigmentation response than dark.
  we recommend: oil-free sunscreens which contain physical (not chemical) filters, so there is less chance of irritation.
- **oriental & asian skin** – has fairly good inbuilt defence: its yellowy pigment and dry tendency makes it dull and line-prone, but it is less likely to go patchy than dark skins and, having more melanin than pale, is better protected from photo-ageing.
  we recommend: sunscreens with hydrating lipids to supplement natural skin oils.

always ...

- Use high factor sunscreens to boost your body's own (limited) natural protection. Wearing sunblock (SPF 30 and higher) is vital when you first go in the sun; after that, don't use lower than SPF10 on your body. Don't worry you will still get a tan because sunscreens don't block out all of the sun. SPF2, for example, blocks out about 50 per cent of UVB rays (the ones that make you go brown), while SPF10 blocks out about 85 per cent.
- Ideally, wear broadspectrum sunscreens which filter out UVA *and* UVB. If sunscreen doesn't contain zinc oxide or titanium dioxide it doesn't give UVA defence so is *not* broadspectrum and not worth wearing.
- Wear water-resistant sunscreens – they have the same SPF value after 40 minutes in the water.

never ...

- Lie on a sunbed – not even when you are wearing sunscreen: sunbeds blast you with intense UV rays (a 20-minute session can be equal to – and as damaging as – a day unprotected on a tropical beach) which massively increases the risk of skin cancer. It doesn't 'prepare' you for the beach because your natural protection is only *ever* equal to SPF2 in sunscreen; being brown doesn't mean you are less likely to burn.

- Allow yourself to burn: sunburn is a repair process – it's your body's way of trying to mend the damage that has been caused and this is why your skin is inflamed. Beauty products can soothe skin but they can't cure a burn or completely reverse sun damage.
- Use a factor lower than SPF15 on your face or – if you are balding – your head.

shopping for sunscreens

Before you head for the shops or flash your cash:

1. Make sure you know what level of protection (that means which SPF numbers) you need.
2. If you want the best protection you can get, make sure the sunscreen gives broadspectrum protection from UVA *and* UVB rays. If it hasn't got avobenzone, titanium dioxide or zinc oxide on its ingredient list you are not even getting half the protection you should be no matter how high the SPF number.
3. Decide whether you want cream, lotion, gel or spray – each has their own advantages, but sprays are especially handy for applying to wriggling children.

... sunscreens we rate:

Julia Caudalie Vinosun Anti Ageing Sun Cream SPF25 (£27 for 40ml): 'I'd never use anything under SPF20 on my face or body, especially since I've got a bit of high colour, and this sunscreen is light but still gives my rosy cheeks heavyweight protection.'

Kate Sisley Broadspectrum Sunscreen SPF40 (£52 for 40ml) and Caudalie Vinosun Anti-Ageing Sun Cream SPF25: 'Space is guaranteed in my suitcase for these two every year, as well as Clarins Oil-Free Sun Care Spray SPF15 (£15 for 150ml): it works upside-down and doesn't need rubbing in – too much effort when it's really hot.'

the 8 best sunscreens

the mission to find you the most user-friendly sunscreens on the market.

the criteria our testers judged the sunscreens they tried on their efficacy not their screening performance or ability to prevent skin from burning as we feel that this is entirely subjective. So our testers did not rate products for how well they protected them from the sun. They judged products on factors like how easy they were to apply (i.e. if they were sprays they had to work upside-down so you could apply them to the backs of your legs – you would be amazed at how many don't), how comfortable they were to wear and what they smelled like.

Clarins Sun Block Stick For Sensitive Areas £11 for 5gm

'This sunscreen was made with me in mind,' said Louise (34). 'I can't bear creams – they get all sandy and horrible, so its twist-up mechanism is perfect because it stays clean.' We think this is probably best for an active person because it slips easily into a pocket or wear it around your neck for easy access. Its texture is similar to lip balm (solid) and although it has good slip factor – so you can apply it easily to your skin or just isolated bits like your nose or shoulders – it isn't greasy and it absorbs quickly. 'It went on well, and it's great for skiers because you can hang it round your neck. I'd definitely recommend it to my sportier friends,' said Alice (34).

the science bit: water- and sweat-resistant, it contains Clarins' unique sun care complex Sunactyl, which aims to support the skin's own protective abilities, and moisturisers like shea butter and sesame and almond oils. Available in SPF30.

Dermalogica Solar Defence Booster £23.60 for 30ml

One of those products that, once tried many seem to get hooked on. 'It has a lovely smell of lavender,' said Sue (51). 'And I liked the fact that I could mix it with my moisturiser or foundation and wear them together – it means you really can wear it all year round. Most sunscreens are far too thick and sticky for that I think. I wish I'd known about it before.'

the science bit: contains avobenzone so provides broadspectrum defence from UVA and UVB rays, and includes grape seed extract, green tea and vitamins A, E and C – all potent antioxidants which are added to offset some of the sun's ageing damage. Available in SPF30 (but if you mix it with your moisturiser or foundation the SPF rating goes down to 17).

Sisley Botanical Body Sun Cream £57 for 200ml

'This is the smell of the south of France,' said Lucy (41). 'I absolutely love Sisley sunscreens – apart from smelling gorgeous, they are incredibly easy to wear absorbing quickly and smoothing onto your skin easily.' Victoria (37) tried various sunscreens on different members of her family for *Beauty Scoop* but kept this one for herself because she loved it so much. 'It was by far the best one I tried,' she said. 'It's a good effective sunscreen, and although it's got a lovely rich creamy texture it still absorbed well into my skin without leaving white streaks all over me.'

the science bit: enriched with moisturising and 'anti-drying' properties, plus ingredients which aim to strengthen the skin's own photo-protective abilities and geranium essential oil, which acts as an insect repellent. Available in SPF10.

Nivea Sun Children's Sun Spray

£12.85 for 200ml

Children are probably the best guineau pigs for sunscreens you can have – they wriggle, fidget, jump in and out of water, get covered in sand and run around: what better road test could you have? 'It's so easy to apply – it's a really good spray that doesn't break down or stop no matter what angle you're holding the bottle,' said Mel (37). 'But I think the best thing about it is its colour – it's green, so you can see where you have applied it until the colour fades. A brainwave for kids.' 'It's a spray but it's like a light milk,' said Victoria (37), mother of two active boys. 'I felt totally assured that they were protected though. When they ran by me I kept trying to squirt them with it because of its colour.'

the science bit: contains a broadspectrum (UVA and UVB) filter, hydrating glycerine and is water-resistant. Available in SPF20 and 30.

Reimann P20

£11.95 for 100ml

There is quite a cult following for this sun cream – a couple of our testers said they didn't want to try other sunscreens for us because they use nothing but this brand on holiday. Its unique selling point is that it only needs applying once a day – or so Reimann claim – and the only drawback to it (probably because it is so resilient) is that it tends to absorb into your skin quite slowly. 'I backpacked around Central America wearing it,' said Dean (40). 'And it was one of – if not *the* – best travelling companions I took with me, mainly because it's so low maintenance.' Debbie (33) was one of our testers who found that it took time to absorb. But she said it did the job without making her skin feel greasy or clogged up.

the science bit: includes the active ingredient p-aminobenzoic acid (vitamin H) which is what makes it cling so well to your skin. It should be applied at least 90 minutes before you go in the sun (to give it a chance to absorb and bind), and onto clean, unmoisturised skin. Available in SPF** [missing info]

Origins Silent Treatment

£22 for 100ml

Origins' take on sunbathing is refreshing: they realise that sunlight makes us feel better about life, but that sunburn is a bad thing. 'I didn't realise Origins made sunscreens', said Julie (34), 'I'm really impressed! It's a nice facial sunscreen. Not greasy or too thick, so easy to apply; no obvious smell and it lasted well. I still had a lot left over at the end of my holiday'.

the science bit: contains a non-chemical filter – titanium dioxide, and soothing botanical extracts. Available in SPF15.

Lancaster Vitalizing Sun Anti-Ageing Cream £17.50 for 50ml

Several of our testers said this would be the sun care brand they would buy if money was no object. Lancaster is a well-established brand, and everything about the sunscreens smacks of luxury – from the packaging to the feel of the products. Iona (47), who has an olive complexion but always protects her skin in the sun, said 'If I hadn't known Lancaster was an expensive brand I would have known it was a quality product as soon as I put it on my face: it absorbed easily – no white blobs or streaks – and it smells lovely. It's like an expensive face cream and I didn't feel as I was cooking my skin.'

the science bit: enriched with ingredients to aid tanning and damage limitation – it has bio-melanin in it, Lancaster's own protection complex, plus free radical scavengers and softening D-panthenol. Available as SPF15 and 35.

Vichy Capital Soleil Sun Screen Spray £12 for 125ml

Another handy sunscreen spray which Lisa (42) took on her family holiday and made everyone use – for the benefit of *Beauty Scoop*! 'My two kids wore it, my husband and myself,' she said. 'And everyone loved it because it's easy to apply, not at all sticky or greasy, and reassuring because we felt we were all getting proper protection.' If you suffer from heat rash or other sensitivity in the sun this would be a good sunscreen to try because it is very light (so doesn't clog up your pores – one way to sensitise skin in the sun) and fragrance-free.

the science bit: contains antioxidant vitamin E and thermal water from the Vichy spa in France to soothe skin and prevent irritation. Available in SPF40.

aftersun products

Is there any point in splashing out on special aftersun products when you could just use good old body lotion? Good question! And we would be the first to tell you if there wasn't a need. But the answer is actually yes, there is logic to using specific aftersun gels, sprays and creams.

Now before you start thinking that aftersun can undo all the bad things the sun has done to your skin during the day, stop: it doesn't. *No product can*. The deal you get with the sun is a lovely tan, but irreversibly damaged (that means aged) skin, and the damage honestly does catch up with you in the end; sunbathing is like making a pact with the devil.

Good aftersuns though are specially formulated to make your tan last longer and enhance the way it looks with a tan. They aim to regenerate your skin, partially offset the damage (they are packed with the right ingredients to do this) caused by the sun. So you could say that they are worth their weight in gold, especially when you consider how much time and 'effort' goes into honing a sun-kissed body.

There are, as ever, some great aftersuns and some bad ones. Read on to find out which are worthy of your hard-earned cash.

what makes a good aftersun?

1. **a light texture**: even though you imagine thick aftersuns are going to do more for your skin, it's better to go for one with a lighter texture because it hydrates your skin without suffocating it or trapping heat in the tissues which can damage skin further.
2. **one that doesn't make too many claims**: remember that aftersun *cannot* reverse the damage you have done to your skin during exposure. It can only re-nourish it and soothe it. Don't be taken in by aftersuns that claim to be anti-ageing.
3. **good application**: like sunscreen, aftersun should dispense efficiently. For instance, if it's a spray it should spray upside-down so you can get it on the backs of your legs and arms; if it doesn't it's a gimmick.

shopping for aftersuns

Before you head for the shops or flash your cash:

1. Decide whether you want spray, cream or gel: each has its own bonuses.
2. Decide whether you need an aftersun for sensitive skin.
3. Work out how much you will need: there is no point wasting money on a bumper-size bottle of the stuff when you are only going on a week's holiday.
4. Decide how much you want to spend: our testers reported success with both competitively-priced and expensive brands.

... aftersuns we rate:

Julia Badger Bali Balm Soothing After Sun Care (£5.99 for 2oz): 'I haven't burned badly for years, but this product – as well as other aloe vera-based creams – is best for cooling skin down after being in the sun.'

Kate Clarins After Sun Replenishing Moisture Care (£21.50 for 50ml): 'Perfect texture, perfect smell, but the best thing about this product is the way it dispenses the cream from a hole in its top – so you never waste it, it never gets sand in it or gunky around the lid.'

the best 2 aftersuns

the mission to find the most effective, user-friendly aftersuns on the market.

the criteria our testers judged the aftersuns they tried on their ability to moisturise, soothe and cool their skin; they also took a view on whether or not the aftersuns they tried enhanced their tans – which some of them now claim to do – how they smelled, how easy they were to apply and how comfortable to wear.

Lancaster Tan Maximiser Soothing Moisturizer (Face)

£18 for 50ml

Despite its rather ambitious claims, this aftersun got 10/10 from two of our testers who said it matched our testing criteria perfectly. 'I thought it worked beautifully,' said Laura (35). 'I used it at the end of each day and I'm sure my tan lasted longer than normal. I have fair skin and don't tan that deeply – so what colour I do get I like to hold on to!' 'It was lovely to use – that's probably why it costs a bit more, has no real smell, is very hydrating and soothing,' said Allie (45). 'What more do you want from an aftersun?'

the science bit: a reparative and hydrating formula which contains a complex called Heliotan – a blend of amino acids, caffeine and trace elements – which Lancaster claim 'accelerates' the production of melanin in the body.

Neal's Yard Remedies Aloe Vera Cooling Spray

£6.50 for 100ml

Two of our testers said they thought it was 'magic' because it provided an instant fix for sunburn. Jill (58) said, 'It's a lovely refreshing spray and worked wonders on my shoulders, which I burned. It's got a lovely fragrance too – lavender I think – and it was immediately cooling, which was truly wonderful on the red bits.' Maria (27) said, 'It was very moisturising, excellent for a spray product.' Another tester said she would buy it because it comes in a light, plastic bottle that makes more sense for travelling.

the science bit: contains soothing and hydrating aloe vera and lavender essential oil, both superb natural remedies for red, over-cooked skin.

BODY CARE

Is there a smooth, toned, hair-free and manicured body under your jeans, t-shirt and trainers waiting to be confidently shown off to the rest of the world this summer? We thought so!

The problem is usually time. We can be so diligent about looking after our hair and faces – the parts that are on show. But most of don't give the rest of our bodies anywhere near the same attention because we think we don't have time to go through the motions on a daily basis, so there is no point doing it at all – or at least until it's essential.

If this is you, listen up: the beauty of body care – exfoliation, moisturising and depilation – is that most of it doesn't need anything like the rigid frequency of skin care. Unless you are trying to improve the tone and profile of your figure with active contouring or cellulite treatments (which does need daily attention), you can get away with tending your body a few times a week for a few minutes. And we reckon this approach is a whole lot healthier than being a slave to the local beauty salon or locking yourself in the bathroom for a couple of hours and trying to 'recreate' a spa experience. Sorry, but who does this?!

We think the most practical and successful approach to body care is to set your own agenda: give yourself as much time as you can (don't forget it's good for your mind as well as your body), don't feel guilty because you are not constantly charging off to try the latest beauty treatment, and buy high-performance products that fit into your life style.

On the following pages we will show you how to achieve this ideal.

What you will find out about in this chapter:

- Whether products which claim to reduce excess hair growth actually work
- Why most of us have still got cellulite despite the mountain of 'remedies'
- Why body lotion is a seriously underrated beauty product
- How much more body exfoliator can do for you than just make your skin smooth

body moisturisers

According to our survey, these are the main reasons why so many of you don't bother with body lotion:

1. You can't afford it: lots of you said that if you had more money to spend on beauty you would buy body moisturisers – and luxury ones, as so many of you said that the feelgood factor is as important as the product's performance.
2. You haven't got time: nearly everyone we sent a survey to said they don't have time to wait for it to absorb before getting dressed or going to bed.
3. You can't bear overpowering scent: understandably none of you likes the idea of walking around all day feeling a bit – well – *slimy*, and smelling synthetic. You like body moisturisers to be light and fresh (or undetectable) – the reason many of you use Johnson's Baby Lotion.
4. Your body is normally covered with clothes: what is the point when no one can see the rough goose-pimply skin on your upper arms and your dry, scaly shins?

To be honest, if those reasons sound familiar you are either using the wrong product or are deluded into thinking that your body can survive without any upkeep.

Most of the skin on your body is thicker than your face, so it would be fair to say it has a greater level of resilience. And it is usually clothed, so unlike your face it is protected from ageing ultraviolet (UV) light and pollution. But it will still benefit from body lotion, which – as well as moisturising – can work wonders on the tone and texture of your skin and ultimately improve the way your overall body looks.

'how much body moisturiser should you use? Lots of our testers asked this and we say slosh it on – you can never over-moisturise your body'

We are not promising that you will look like one of those pubescent models on telly who would not know what slack or goose-pimply skin was if it hit them in the face, and obviously we realise that because you have a life some things have to give and body lotion is a low priority. But even if you only apply it a few times a week you are less likely to have those last-minute 'look at the state of my arms/legs/back/chest!' panics before putting on a swimsuit or skimpier clothing.

Body lotion is very clever these days. Some do much more than moisturise, they actively make skin smoother and firmer, and believe us, having supple, smooth and plump skin goes a long way to improving the look of your whole body.

why body moisturiser is a good thing

- It hydrates your skin which makes a visible difference to the way it looks (especially helpful over cellulite areas) – now and in the future. By keeping skin supple it may prevent (not erase) stretchmarks.
- It makes skin smoother and softer – again bonuses which help its overall look – especially if it contains alpha hydroxy acids (AHAs) which continually exfoliate skin (see more about AHAs in the chapter on skin care on page 18).
- If it's applied properly (i.e. massaged in well whenever you use it) it promotes your circulation and natural cleansing processes, which can prevent a build-up of fluid retention and cellulite.
- It can make your skin firmer and more toned – only superficially – but again this improves the look of your whole body.
- If it contains light-reflective particles – which bounce light in a flattering way off your skin – it makes it shimmer (without being greasy), look younger and healthier, and enhances a tan.

how to apply body moisturiser

And you thought all you had to do was smother yourself in it?! As with most beauty products the way you apply body moisturiser is part of the key to its effectiveness. French women give their legs a mini massage everyday when they apply body or anti-cellulite creams because they know how effective this is at keeping the circulation and lymph ticking over (and how important this is to their health, body shape and skin condition) which helps prevent any fluid retention. If you can put aside 15 minutes every other day – or even just twice a week – to do the following massage with body lotion you will be doing yourself a lot more favours than just moisturising your skin:

> 'can't be bothered to moisturise? Add some nourishing oils to a warm bath instead (but don't stay in it too long or you will defeat the object)'

1. Apply body lotion to your hands and warm it up between your palms. Start by rubbing it into your feet, and use your fist to knead your soles and massage upper edge of arches with thumbs to stimulate your kidneys.
2. Use your thumb to massage the skin around your anklebone and push up behind anklebone into calves.
3. Drag your thumbs up the backs of your calves to the backs of your knees in lines to promote lymph and circulation – you are literally pushing fluids back up your legs. Use your thumbs to massage the fleshy insides of knees (this can be sensitive), and knead the backs of your knees with a fist.
4. Push your thumbs up the front of your thighs in lines from knees to groin.
5. Massage outer thighs with both hands, kneading to break up stubborn fat deposits and promote circulation which can be sluggish here.

do 'spa' moisturisers work better?

It's only a three-letter word, but 'spa' has huge clout when it comes to giving beauty products (especially body care products like moisturisers) credibility. So what exactly does it mean – that your body moisturiser is better than regular non-spa versions? That it's more *natural*? Not necessarily. In fact, rarely. Spa-based products fall into two categories: those that are no different whatsoever to regular beauty products except that they might have a manufactured oceanic scent or sea-blue tint, and those that come from genuine spas (usually in France or Italy) and are made with real sea extracts like seasalt and seaweed that can have potent conditioning and cleansing properties. Unfortunately, the word 'spa' is as misused as the words 'aromatherapy' and 'detox' now. So if you are thinking of buying into the concept of 'marine benefits' do your homework and find out where the product came from first.

'how often should you apply body moisturiser? Lots of you asked this in our survey, and in an ideal world you would do it after every bath. But we know that is unrealistic, so we think you should aim for two or three times a week, and you should see a clear difference in the appearance of your skin within a week'

shopping for body moisturisers:

Before you head for the shops or flash your cash:

1. Decide what kind of body moisturiser you want – one that simply moisturises your skin, one that has toning and smoothing properties or all three? It really helps to narrow the choice down. If you go for a body oil, think about whether you want a dry or regular oil – the latter makes you much more shiny.
2. Think about smell: do you want to smell like the moisturiser you are about to try? (And if you can't test the smell don't buy it).
3. Consider your life style: if you think you have not got time to apply body lotion everyday would a quick moisturising spray be more practical for you?
4. Decide how much you want to spend: as you will see from the responses we got from our testers, you don't have to fork out to get a decent body moisturiser because the budget brands perform very well. If you do splash out on a more expensive cream though don't keep it for 'best': lots of the people who did our survey admitted they only use expensive products occasionally to justify the expense. But you get the best results when you use products regularly.

... body moisturisers we rate:

Julia Chantecaille Frangipani Body Cream (£59 for 200ml): 'Pure indulgence, and if I could always afford to use it I would. It smells gorgeous, sinks into your skin quickly and makes it fabulously soft. Jo Malone's body lotions always go on my Christmas list too. I'm obsessive about moisturising, but not faithful to one brand because I think using anything is better than nothing and the cheaper brands are as good at moisturising as the expensive ones.'

Kate I Coloniali Deep Massage Body Cream with Myrrh (£27.50 for 200ml): 'I'm an all-or-nothing girl when it comes to body cream – I either apply it religiously everyday or don't bother for weeks. This is the one I always go back to. I just think it's been made by a genius. It hydrates and exfoliates – the buffing grains melt as you rub it in – so your skin gets a double softening whammy.'

the 7 best body moisturisers

the mission To find you the most effective and user-friendly body moisturisers on the market.

the criteria Our testers judged the body moisturisers on their ability to hydrate, soften and smooth their skin; improve their skin tone; absorb fast; how comfortable they felt to wear and their smell.

Nivea Body Firming Lotion Q10

£5.49 for 200ml

Easily the most popular of all the body moisturisers we roadtested. 'FANTASTIC VALUE FOR MONEY,' wrote Jackie (28) and Lucy (32) in block capitals on their questionnaires. 'It's not greasy and quickly absorbs into your skin,' said Jackie (37). 'It honestly made my skin look different,' wrote Kari (41), and then scribbled it out and wrote 'much better!'.

the science bit: Q10 is an enzyme found naturally in our cells and Nivea say that when added to a cream it firms skin and kick-starts cellular activity, which slows down with age.

Vaseline Essential Moisture

£1.99 for 200ml

Our testers loved this cream because of its no-nonsense image and brilliant hydrating qualities. Saba (31) said: 'I give it ten out of ten because it does what it says it will – nothing very fancy. It just moisturises your skin, yet it doesn't feel "heavy", which is how I imagine a good moisturiser to feel. Great value for money.'

the science bit: All the major hydrating ingredients are packed into this cream – petrolatum emollient oil, panthenol, vitamin E and natural moisturising factors like urea, which help to trap moisture in your skin. It also contains vitamin A, a potent skin smoother.

Body Shop Body Butter

£10 for 200ml

Body Shop's range of differently scented Body Butters came out very well in our road tests with several testers singling out their favourites as olive and mango. Shauna (33) loved the mango 'flavour', and Lucy (41) loved olive. She said, 'It's got a good creamy consistency that really softens up dry areas like your elbows and shins, and it smells ever-so-slightly Mediterranean, but it's nothing too clingy or overpowering.'

the science bit: There are eight different body butters – brazil nut, shea, coconut, sesame, grape seed, olive, mango, melon seed and papaya – each of which has its own benefit on your skin.

Ren Wild Yam Omega 7 Body Repair Cream
£28.95 for 250ml

'I just couldn't fault this product,' says Sam (40). 'It really is amazing – everything from the packaging to the cream's performance is great. My mum loves it, too. I think its main bonus is its softening effect on your skin because its scent isn't really detectible, but it absorbs quickly and it looks great in my bathroom!'

the science bit: The main ingredient is wild yam – which Ren were first to use in a beauty product because they say it can improve skin elasticity, suppleness and smoothness. It also contains sea buckthorn berry oil, said to regenerate skin.

Marks & Spencer Spa Life Moisturising Body Whip
£6 for 200ml

Despite its name – which suggests that by using it you will experience non-specific spa effects – and its scent (an acquired taste) this moisturiser was a huge success. Sarah (34) commented on a marked improvement to her skin: 'It genuinely felt much softer,' she said. 'My boyfriend thought I smelt of a Thai stir-fry, very gingery, and although not very spa-like, in the end we decided we really liked the fragrance.'

the science bit: The key to this formula is a moisturising seaweed extract, but the cream also contains glycerine, a potent moisturiser and protective agent.

Liz Earle Nourishing Botanical Body Cream
£6.50 for 50ml

Rich – it needs to be properly massaged in – but very effective and ideal for anyone with sensitive skin. Joanna (42) described its fragrance as being like 'flowers on a hot sunny day', while Lucy (41) said applying it feels like you are bathing in liquid satin: 'It's wonderfully rich and soft like non-greasy margarine, you can just feel it doing your skin good.'

the science bit: Ingredients include shea butter and vitamin E – popular skin hydrators – plus essential oils lavender, geranium and orange.

Decleor Vitarome
£42.75 for 50ml

The queen of body creams, it offers you every conceivable benefit: 'I can't fault it,' says Dawn (59). 'I defy anyone to; this is how a dream body cream should feel and behave. It's rich and nourishing, but because it's like an emulsion, it's not sticky. It melts into your skin. It's got a light smell. And it makes your skin look amazing. Shame I've found it really because I'm always going to want it now!'

the science bit: as well as moisturisers, this cream contains light reflective pigments – which are the reason why it makes your skin look instantly better (especially if you have got a tan), because they reflect light off your skin in a flattering way and give it a healthy warm glow.

exfoliators

What, you asked in our surveys, is the point of body exfoliators – especially ones that cost more than a fiver? Surely they are not *that much* of a beauty priority?

Well, while we are the first to admit that there are a number of beauty products in existence that the world could do without (neck creams, eyelash primers, face 'slimming' creams, eyeliner tape – who buys this stuff?), body buffers do have a real place in your bathroom cabinet. And if you have ever used a decent one you will know why.

The benefits of a good body scrub can be likened to the way your skin looks and feels after you have been swimming in the sea on holiday: soft, toned, pink and ALIVE! As well being full of minerals which benefit your skin, seawater is rich in salt, so it's a natural exfoliant. That is why your skin feels softer after a dip in it. The gentle abrasive action (and the cool temperature) of the sea also galvanises your circulation, which sends freshly-oxygenated blood rushing up to the skin's surface. This is what makes it look pink, and feel slightly firmer and smoother.

We believe this is what a good exfoliator should do for you: wake your skin (and you) up, promote circulation and make your body soft, plump, supple and pink. Perhaps it is something you need to experience?

when to use a body exfoliator

As well as making your skin feel softer because it buffs off dead, flaky bits of skin, regular exfoliation also increases the rate at which skin cells renew themselves, and one theory is that this can delay premature ageing because it strengthens cellular activity and the 'cement' that binds cells together. Aside from that, skin that has just been exfoliated absorbs moisturiser more quickly. Do it once a week if you can – you *will* quickly notice a difference in the look and feel of your skin – and at these times:

- before applying self-tan and going on a holiday in the sun – to shift dead skin before you get a tan (so it doesn't fall off when you have got it)
- before applying anti-cellulite treatments to increase absorption (but remember that no amount of scrubbing or body-brushing will shift one dimple by itself)
- before wearing a low-cut or backless top or dress (but remember to exfoliate chest skin gently because it's very fine)

when not to use a body exfoliator

- when skin is irritated or trying to heal, or on areas where there is psoriasis, eczema or dermatitis
- before getting on the plane home from your holiday in the sun (you should be doing your best to 'stick' your skin – and tan – on before spending hours in an air-conditioned airplane, not buffing it off)
- when you are using a body moisturiser with chemical exfoliants alpha or beta hydroxy acids (AHAs and BHAs) in it – no one's skin needs this much exfoliation
- immediately before or after using a depilatory or hair removal product

shopping for body exfoliators

Before you head for the shops or flash your cash:

1. Decide what kind of exfoliator you want: one which foams up and can be rinsed-off like body cleansing wash, or a water-soluble cream.
2. Check out the smell. As our testers told us, fragrance matters, and if you don't like it you won't use the product – no matter how well it performs.
3. Make sure the exfoliating grains are fine – particles from fruit shells are too big and can scratch your skin – and are dense enough. There is nothing worse than an exfoliator with too few grains in it – a total waste of time and money!
4. Decide how much you want to spend: our testers' responses proved that you can get good buffers from both budget and top-end brands, but you tend to pay more for one with a better quality scent.

... body moisturisers we **rate:**

Julia Elemis Exotic Lime & Ginger Salt Glow (£32.50 for 14.5oz): 'I love the smell and the grittiness of the salt – and the fact that it doesn't make my bath grimey. It also leaves a light coat of moisturising oil on your skin.'

Kate Hardys Frangipani Salt Scruff (£19.95 for 750gm): 'I think this is a dream body exfoliator: it's scented with one of my favourite smells, it's got lots of big seasalty flakes in it and it leaves your skin smooth and soft because it's not drying.'

the 6 best body exfoliators

the mission To find you the most effective and user-friendly body exfoliators on the market.

the criteria Our testers judged the body exfoliators they tried on their ability to make skin feel softer and more supple (lots of our testers say they have had bad experiences with coarse exfoliators that have left their skin gasping for cream), on the density of their buffing particles and their smell.

Origins Salt Rub £25 for 600gm

We are both big fans of salt scrubs because sea salt is naturally rich in minerals, and the 'flakes' buff well without being hard and dissolve in water, so you don't get that vile brown ring around the bath after you have used it and rinsed it off. Polly (19) said this one 'smells so fresh and works so well it gives you a real kick start in the morning. I felt so much more alive – warmer too, and I felt like going to work'.

the science bit: The Dead Sea salts are suspended in a nourishing oily base made from macadamia nuts, sweet almonds and soybean, and the formula also includes invigorating spearmint and rosemary essential oils.

Body Shop Papaya Body Scrub £10 for 200ml

You have got to like sweet smelling products to like this as the papaya content in this scrub certainly has a strong presence. Shauna (33) is one of the testers who loved it – she thinks it is 'so delicious it's good enough to eat', which is lucky because she also noted that 'it really lasts'. She said the scrub is a hard worker, too – without being too harsh on your skin in the way that some body exfoliators can be.

the science bit: This exfoliator doesn't contain papaya by accident. The fruit has an enzyme in it called papain, which is a natural exfoliant, so it dissolves keratin, a hard protein found in the dead cells you are buffing off. So the old top layer of your skin gets a double buffing whammy.

Fresh Brown Sugar Body Polish £47 for 435gm

Sue (40) thinks this body buffer is a miracle, commenting 'my skin felt fantastic (underlined several times) after using it and I didn't need to moisturise afterwards because there was no tightness. I can't believe the sensation – you've got the coarseness of the sugar and smoothness of the oils, and the combination is out of this world'. It has a strong scent, so you need a sweet tooth to enjoy it: Paula (24) said, 'The scrubbing bits are sugar grains and work so well although it's weird buffing with something that smells this good.'

the science bit: The buffing particles – pure brown sugar – are in a base of more than 20 oils including sweet almond, evening primrose, passiflora (which boosts your circulation) and arnica, so this is a very luxurious product.

Borghese Salt Scrub

£30 for 455gm

Its name suggests it is one thing (gritty and salty) but it feels like something quite different because the buffing grains are so fine – more like marble dust really. So as Heather (31) pointed out, 'It's brilliant for people like me who have dry and sometimes sensitive skin. I find most exfoliators too much – they're too lumpy and grind into your skin. But I loved this because it's got a creamy texture, so it almost feels like you're rubbing a soft paste into your skin, but it still exfoliates and sends your dead skin down the plug hole. Full marks.'

the science bit: The magic ingredient is Borghese's aqua de vita complex – spa water extracted from Italy's Montecatini spa, which is full of skin conditioning minerals. It also contains mango and shea butter, olive and grape seed oils.

Boots Mediterranean Mandarin, Lime & Orange Invigorating Body Scrub

£5.25 for 250ml

Bit of a mouthful for a body scrub, but our tester Victoria (37) said, 'It's the best if you're on a budget but want an exfoliator which has enough grit to it, and this one has just the right amount of "scratch".' She gave it top marks, but wavered a bit over the scent when she first used it, describing it as being 'like a sweet fizzy drink, but it turns into a soft scent afterwards which I actually liked'.

the science bit: The buffing bits in this wash-off peach coloured buffer is sweet orange peel – which is softer than the particles in many exfoliators.

Circaroma Cedarwood, Lemongrass & Basil Body Scrub

£13 for 350gm

Sophie (30) thinks this is one of the most 'heavenly' beauty products she has ever used. 'You get the right amount of rough – it buffs your skin without making it sting or smart, and the luxury of a really smooth oil to nourish your skin afterwards. I liked the fact that I didn't have to use any body lotion after it, and its fragrance is out of this world.' Kerry (39) added 'it's not at all harsh on your skin – good if it's sensitive like mine – and it smells delicious.'

the science bit: Enriched with organic essential oils like orange, basil – which has antiseptic qualities – cedarwood, lemongrass and cajeput.

foot care

You either love feet or hate them. Leonardo da Vinci loved them – he thought they were masterpieces of engineering and works of art. Neither of us are big fans, frankly – we think our toes look like cocktail sausages and both of us have thick ankles.

Leonardo had a point though. Each foot has 26 bones, 114 ligaments and 20 finely-tuned muscles – the mechanics that allow us to stand upright and walk. On this point alone feet deserve a break and a bit of TLC every so often. Think about it: they support your entire weight *day-in-day-out*, they're often crammed into shoes that don't fit properly because you HAD TO HAVE the shoes, and they are prone to delights like calluses, bunions, corns, blisters and athlete's foot (so vile). And if you get away without having any of these complaints – ever – you are very lucky.

'the trend for foot surgery – having liposuction on your ankles or the bone shaved – so they look better in expensive sandals is beauty at its most mad (and sad)'

Feet are also challenged in the looks department. They're not the prettiest things in the world to look at (unless they happen to be in a pair of Manolo Blahniks), and they tend to get dry and flaky around the heels, which is never a good look.

But like your body, the amazing thing about feet is that often the simplest treatment – even just massaging them with moisturiser – can make a marked difference to their overall appearance and how you feel about them and yourself.

how to resuscitate your feet

A foot massage can be a tonic for your whole body. Try this little routine whenever you have a bit of time to yourself:

1. Warm plenty of foot cream or balm between your palms (don't hesitate to slosh loads of the stuff on), then apply it lightly over both feet.
2. Use your fist to knead your soles and your thumbs to massage the upper edge of the arches of your feet to stimulate your kidneys.
3. Use your thumb to massage the skin around your anklebone and push up behind anklebone into calves.
4. Push both thumbs together up the front of each foot in lines to help clear any puffiness from fluid retention.

how to deal with boring foot problems

- **Post-shopping, pre-menstrual or pregnant feet** (i.e. swollen and puffy): shower them with cold water, then follow the massage guidelines above using a foot cream containing cooling ingredients such as menthol and peppermint, lie flat on the floor and rest your feet up against the wall at right angles to allow trapped fluids to run back up your legs.
- **Cold feet**: use the showerhead to spray your legs and feet with hot and cold blasts of water – it helps to kickstart your circulation. (When Kate has really cold feet she sticks them in a bowl of hot water mixed with mustard powder. She says it smells so awful it makes your eyes water but it works.)
- **Shoe obsessive's feet** (i.e. recurring corns): don't buy shoes that don't fit no matter how gorgeous because chafing causes corns.
- **Itchy feet**: athlete's foot can drive you NUTS – the itching is enough to send you round the bend. If you get it you should stop wearing trainers day-in-day-out (they make your feet hot which the fungus that is athlete's foot loves, especially when it's sweaty between the toes, too), properly dry your feet after a bath, dust between your toes with powder and don't walk around barefoot or the rest of the household will get it.

shopping for foot products

Before you head for the shops or flash your cash:

1. Decide whether you need a foot cream. This might sound mad coming from two beauty journalists who have spent over six months road testing hundreds of products, but we have not done this just to make you buy products you don't need. If your feet are dry, swollen or sore you would benefit from a foot cream – and ideally one containing cooling and soothing ingredients such as menthol. Otherwise, use regular body lotion.
2. Decide how much you want to spend: none of the foot care products our testers rated cost the earth.

'to soften the hard skin on your heels and soles soak your feet for ten minutes in a bowl of warm water mixed with a few drops of olive oil'

... foot products we rate:

Julia Philosophy Footnotes Pumice Foot Scrub (£11 for 15gm) 'Total bliss. It's a greeny goo with invigorating menthol in it and if you dig deep enough into the pot you find a thick layer of gritty pumice to rub on your heels and other hard skin areas. I feel like a kid when I use it. It's so much fun and it works so well.'

Kate Rose & Co Apothecary Tea Tree & Cypress Foot Cream (£5.99 for 30gm): 'My feet really puff up when it's hot so I've done my research and worked my way through most of the cooling foot creams on the market, and this is the one that works the best for me. It's magic.'

the 5 best foot care products

the mission To find you the most effective and user-friendly foot care products on the market.

the criteria Our testers judged the foot care products they tried on their ability to moisturise and soften their skin, absorb quickly and cool their feet. They also took the products' fragrance into consideration.

Boots Mediterranean Foot Butter £4.75 for 200ml

Joanna (42) thought this 'smelled like an Italian deli – delicious'. Her big foot problem is dry skin and this was her litmus test for this product. It passed. 'It worked wonders,' she said. Juliet (23) said, 'It's such a pleasant cream it makes putting foot cream on less of a chore. It's not too thick either, so it actually goes in. It must be one of those great budget buys.'

the science bit: This is a very simple – and very Mediterranean – formula which includes olive oil, lemon and invigorating thyme extract.

Sixtus Alpine Herbs Foot Balsam £10.95 for 50ml

After using this product, Kate (32) wrote, 'Even my physiotherapist commented on the difference!' Her feet are softer, even the hard-skinned bits around her heels, and it seemed to do this with ease. Kate was sent three foot care products (in error) and charitably tried them all for us, but says this is the only one she would buy.

the science bit: The cream is jam-packed with invigorating natural ingredients – mountain thyme, dwarf pine, rosemary, peppermint and reparative lavender, plus Sixtus' special herbal extract formula.

Pedicure Opi Foot Soak Tea Tree Bath

£9.75 for 125ml

Frankly, we can't think of anyone who regularly soaks their feet (which is a shame because foot soaks are very beneficial), but Sandra (41) insists that she has been converted into one of those people by this product. 'It cleans your feet, softens them, makes them cool and refreshed – great on a hot day – and there is the added bonus of having an excuse to sit there and do nothing for ten minutes,' she wrote.

the science bit: The key ingredient in this treatment is tea tree oil – refreshing, antiseptic (it gets rid of itchy athlete's foot), soothing and healing.

Creative Nail Design Spa Pedicure Sea Salt Glow

£8.95 for 5oz

This sexy little purple exfoliator got a great vote of confidence from our testers. 'I never thought I'd get to use an exfoliator on my feet – what luxury,' remarked a happy Lou (51). 'It was a joy to use and my feet haven't looked so good for years. I just want to show them off now.'

the science bit: Good sized chunks of seasalt in a base of sunflower oil, with vitamin E, it gives your feet a bit of rough – and smooth.

Neutrogena Foot Cream

£4.99 for 50ml

'This is just such a good product because a little goes a long, long way,' said Annie (26) a dedicated clubber who admits that her feet often suffer after a night out. 'I needed a decent moisturising cream but my budget doesn't stretch very far so I was really pleased to discover this. It's not greasy and it works a treat. My feet feel softer and working it in really helps to ease aches and pains.'

the science bit: A glycerine-based cream containing vitamin E and skin-softening panthenol.

hand care

Of all the parts of our bodies our hands are probably the most left out – especially when you think how hard they work for us. This is one reason why they age so fast and are so difficult to bring back from the brink once you have let them go.

The other reason they age rapidly is that there are relatively few oil (sebaceous) glands in the skin – certainly compared to the rest of your body anyway – so they get dry, and dry skin is said to age faster. Like your face, your hands are constantly exposed to ultraviolet (UV) light too: there you are, happily driving along in the car, washing up or typing at your desk by a window and the sun's powerful and ageing rays – which go through glass – are busy giving you a pair of wizened old paws.

'an incentive to look after your hands: they reveal your age far more than your face, which is why you need to use protective hand cream if you want to preserve them'

The way to stop your hands from ageing fast (and telling the world that you are older than you are) is to protect and moisturise them as you would your face.

Which means you have to remember to put on hand cream.

We think the world divides into two types when it comes to hand cream: those who use it and those who don't. To be honest, most of us don't have time to keep sloshing the stuff on – UNLESS it goes on easily and sinks into your skin even faster.

Which is where our intrepid testers came in.

how to make your hands look better fast

1. Exfoliate them – a body scrub will do for this job, but if you haven't got one mix some seasalt with a dash of cooking oil and rub that over your hands. Then wash, rinse and dry your hands.
2. Rub hand cream into your hands and nails, very *gently* pushing back the cuticles (not so far that it hurts) as you do it.

your hands love

- moderate temperatures
- hand cream
- massage

your hands hate

- water – especially hot
- drying household detergents
- harsh weather
- unprotected, prolonged exposure to ultraviolet (UV) rays

which hand cream do you need?

- **nourishing creams** do what they suggest: moisturise your hands!
- **barrier creams** may also moisturise hands but also physically protect them from the elements or damaging work such as DIY, washing up (if you don't like wearing gloves) and gardening.
- **protective creams** may also moisturise hands but also contain a filter which protects them from ultraviolet (UV) light. Always buy a UV protective cream which offers *broadspectrum protection*; in other words, defends your skin from UVA *and* UVB rays – both age and damage skin (see our section on sun care on page 59), but not all sunscreens contain filters which screen both types of ray out.

shopping for hand care products

Before you head for the shops or flash your cash:

1. Decide what you want from hand cream – anti-ageing benefits, super-strength nourishment, protection or all three.
2. Work out when you are likely to use hand cream – if it's too rich and greasy it will usually take longer to absorb so you won't want to use it during the day and are better off with a lighter, fast-absorbing formula.
3. Check out the scent. Fragrance really matters; if you don't like it, you won't use the product, no matter how well it works.
4. Decide how much you want to spend: our testers unanimously agreed that more expensive hand creams performed better than the cheapies. Many also said that the feel-good factor of using a luxury hand cream is almost as significant to them as its performance. So money does talk in this case ..

... hand care products we rate:

Julia DiproBase (£12 for 50gm): 'This is a basic emollient you can buy at the chemist, and having used it on my children's little eczema patches I found that it's also very good at softening dry hands. I also love Crabtree & Evelyn La Source Hand Recovery (£12.50 for 100ml), which isn't a conventional hand cream in that it's actually more like a scrub which you apply to dry hands, rub in and rinse off. It softens washing-up-hands beautifully.'

Kate Chantecaille Retinol Hand Cream with Rose & Vitamin C (£52 for 75ml): 'I think this is the Rolls Royce of hand creams. It's got a bit of retinol in it which makes a big difference to the softness of your skin, and it smells divine.

the top 7 hand care products

the mission To find you the most effective and user-friendly hand care products on the market.

the criteria Our testers judged the hand care products they tried on their ability to moisturise and soften hard and dry skin, the speed with which they absorbed into skin and the strength and wearability of their scent.

Neutrogena Norwegian Formula Handcream

£3.69 for 50ml

The best of the cheapies, this concentrated cream works really well on chronically dry hands and any other rough, hard bits you might have. 'It's pretty thick – a sort of gel-like balm, so you have to work it in quite hard, but it's worth the effort,' said Emily (31). 'And I think it's as near-perfect a product as you can get. It works so well and even my nails look better.' Lucy (41) said, 'It lasts such a long time and works immediately: it's as if you have put on a pair of moisturising gloves.'

the science bit: The secret to its formula is glycerine – an ingredient which hydrates the upper layers of your skin and forms a protective barrier over your skin so moisture can't escape; and it contains ten times more of it than any other hand cream on the market. You can buy it scented or unscented.

Gatineau Vitamin A Suractivee Hand Cream

£11.50 for 100ml

Jane (40) was one of the testers who gave this cream full marks because she said, 'It's the first hand cream I've ever used which actually had a visible effect on the age spots on the backs of my hands. It's a lovely rich cream but it doesn't feel greasy. I can see myself using it regularly, which is saying something for a hand cream.'

the science bit: It contains antioxidant vitamins which prevent and may diminish age spots and counteract the effects of free radicals, the molecules that actively age your skin. It also contains a sunscreen and if you apply it more thickly and leave it on for about ten minutes it works as an intense moisturising mask.

Cellex-C Skin Firming Hand Cream

£55 for 50ml

OK OK *calm down* – this one is really expensive, we know, and you will be wondering how on earth a hand cream can justify this kind of price? Our thoughts exactly, until we got our tester replies back, and it seems it can get away with this price tag because every single person who tried it (without knowing how much it costs) said it gave fantastic results. 'A total hand reincarnation,' said Marina (52). 'It's brilliant – what on earth is in it?' asked Philly (35). 'I've never seen my hands look so rested – it's as if I haven't done a day's work in my life.'

the science bit: The magic ingredients in this formula are vitamin C – an antioxidant which increases production of collagen and elastin, the fibres under your skin that keep it firm and springy, tyrosine –which is said to activate skin-tanning melanin, zinc and soothing camomile.

Mary Cohr Youth & Beauty Hand Cream

£9 for 75ml

One tester loved this so much she sent us a note pleading for some more! Kate (42) thinks it is 'a miracle product' (you can't have a better recommendation) that has changed her view of products such as hand cream being a luxury she isn't prepared to fork out for. 'I've got stronger nails which look healthier, my hands are softer and it's just such a pleasure to use this product,' she said.

the science bit: The key ingredients in this cream are amino acids, vitamins and nasturtium extract which is said to soften age spots and even up skin tone; it also contains vitamin B5, the property that strengthens your nails.

Clarins Hand & Nail Treatment

£14 for 100ml

A big favourite with lots of our testers: 'You can see why people love it as it does exactly what it says it will do,' said Caroline (34). 'It moisturises and softens your hands, softens the skin, and hardens your nails so they are flexible not brittle. You don't need a separate nail strengthener. I've still got age spots on the backs of my hands, but they are less noticeable. My hands are a real mess because I ride a lot and don't look after them, so any cream that makes a difference is a real hero as far as I'm concerned.'

the science bit: The main properties are nourishing sesame oil extract, shea butter which forms a protective barrier over skin, Japanese mulberry extract, said to diminish existing age spots, and myrrh, a nail strengthening agent.

Blisslabs Glamour Gloves

Glamour Gloves Gel, £18 for 75ml, Glamour Gloves, £36

Tamsin (28) thought these were some kind of joke when we sent them to her – 'I couldn't believe they were for real,' she wrote, 'they look *so* gimmicky. But I did what I was told – slathered the gel on and put the gloves on – and I have to say I was really impressed by the results: seriously soft hands. I got my mum and sister to try them and we all think they're brilliant. A gimmick, but definitely a good one.'

the science bit: The gel is enriched with mandarin oil, antioxidant vitamin E and glycerine – all moisturising and protective ingredients; it also contains lemon, parsley and mulberry root extact, which make skin smooth and with regular use may reduce age spots. The gloves have a polymer gel lining which is infused with more skin-softeners – grape seed, jojoba and olive oils, and vitamin E.

Skin Wisdom Extra Care Age Defying Hand Cream

£6 for 50ml

Helen (39) thinks she is addicted to this cream. 'Since I tested it for your book I've bought two more tubes of it,' she wrote. 'I've got one by the sink, one in my desk drawer at work and one by the telly sofa. It's *so* good. It sinks in quickly, and I can't believe the difference it's made to my nails. It's so logical for a cream to help your nails and cuticles, I can't believe it's taken me so long to find one though.'

the science bit: Key ingredients are the antioxidant green tea, mulberry extract to even up skin tone, panthenol – which strengthens nails and softens cuticles –and an SPF of 15.

cellulite treatments

Many of the people who took part in our survey didn't want to test cellulite products for us because they said they had been taken in by their claims, and disappointed, too often. Some asked if they really worked. Others simply said 'some of their claims are hard to believe'. And they are right. Many of them make outrageous claims about 'erasing' cellulite for good. Which is simply not possible.

When cellulite was first identified as 'a different kind of fat' (quite recently because up until the 1980s it was still the normal kind) it opened the floodgates for all kinds of remedies and, depressingly, some hardhearted journalism.

Every summer at least a dozen celebrities are exposed as cellulite 'sufferers' when they are photographed in an unforgiving light on the beach in Barbados or the south of France. Cellulite spotting is a national pastime. And even if you are slim with toned muscles you are likely to have it and be all too aware of it. Unless you are very lucky. Or 14 years old. (Which reminds us: isn't it about time those beauty companies who advertise body-refining products on TV hire models who are mature enough to know what it's actually like to have cellulite – or even a bit of flab?)

'isn't it about time that beauty companies who advertise body-refining products on TV hire models who are old enough to know what it's actually like to have cellulite – or even a bit of flab?'

So for the beauty industry, 'discovering' cellulite was like striking gold. And the more hype there is over it – the more pictures of people with dimply thighs in the press and articles on how to 'get rid of it' – the bigger this part of the business gets.

The thing about cellulite though, is that it has a number of triggers – genes, hormones, lack of exercise, fluid retention, lymph flow and circulation – and the degree to which all (or some) of these affect you varies from person to person. So it is just not possible for one cellulite product to 'fit all', and the best you can hope for is an improvement in the look of the overlying skin. This is the healthiest approach to the market and the problem, because when your skin has good clarity and tone (we are not just talking about muscles here, but suppleness and firmness of skin) cellulite looks less obvious and the overall appearance of the area is much better.

We think this is where cellulite products really come into their own – when they work hard to improve the look of skin and lessen the appearance of cellulite. Good ones effectively boost local circulation and drainage, tangibly easing puffiness and congestion; and can smooth away goosepimples and make skin more supple – all benefits which help to offset the appearance of cellulite far beneath the skin.

These are the kind of cellulite products to invest in, not those that claim to erase the problem completely or reshape you. No beauty product can (or should) single-handedly do that. So don't lose heart if you have not yet had success with anti-cellulite products: just readjust your expectations a little and be prepared for a surprise.

how to maximise the effects of cellulite treatments

As we have already said, anti-cellulite products can greatly improve the look of the overlying skin, but *none of them* can singlehandedly erase cellulite. To do this you need to make the following five key changes to your life style (this is what people mean when they say you have to approach cellulite *holistically*) – and maintain them forever, not just until you get bored, or cellulite will come back:

1. **take exercise**: doing activities that stretch and lengthen your muscles rather than bulking them up which, some say, makes cellulite cling on. That rules out step, stairmaster, jogging and aerobics in favour of sprinting, yoga, tennis or squash and rebounding on a trampoline – which is good for your circulation.
2. **drink water**: aim to sip a 1.5 litre bottle of still water (too much sodium goes into water when they add bubbles) throughout the day to flush impurities out of your system before they get a chance to turn into 'unwanted guests'. Volvic is the best because it has the lowest content of dry residue – that is the unidentified properties in the water which may not be so good for your system.
3. **eat clean**: many believe that cellulite is a build-up of toxins and that certain foods (such as sodium-rich or spicy processed foods and caffeine) are thought to make the problem worse so should be avoided as far as possible. From personal experience, a diet that is low in sugar, that maintains body alkalinity – so avoid acid-forming foods like certain fruit and white wine – and separates proteins from starches works best.
4. **avoid caffeine**: it clogs up the lymph and is acid forming. Although some cellulite products contain a form of caffeine because it has diuretic and circulation boosting powers, when taken orally, caffeine (in coffee and tea) is metabolized differently by your body, and can overload your system, often worsening celllulite.
5. **have massage**: it helps to disperse cellulite, but from experience we can tell you that it needs to be as tough as you can bear: the therapist's fingers should dig deep into the fascial tissue to eke toxins out. Most beauty therapists don't apply enough force – and nowhere near the pressure you need on your backside and thighs to do the job well (it is hard work) – so find a *remedial masseur* who does deep tissue massage and have it twice a month. The litmus test for a good masseur is someone who can visibly lift your backside and make it look a size smaller in one session. They do exist, but not usually in beauty salons.

readjust your expectations

Nearly all of the people who took part in our survey and had something to say about cellulite products told us that they were a waste of money because they 'didn't work'. But nine times out of ten this is a case of having too high expectations. Success rests on readjusting (not lowering) your outlook: getting great results from a cellulite product means getting tangibly firmer, smoother skin with better tone and clarity. Not thighs like a pre-pubescent girl (or boy!).

do contouring tablets work?

Like the creams, they can if they form part of a cellulite regime. Magnesium and potassium are antioxidants that help lymph drainage, so look for these ingredients in the products. The best ones contain flavonoids, nutrients found in some vegetables and fruit which strengthen capillaries thus improving poor circulation – one of cellulite's causes. The ones we rate are Oenobiol Aquadrainant Supplements (£16.50) – a great French import (there is a huge choice of drainage products available over-the-counter in France); Elemis Deep Drainage Body Enhancement Capsules (£19) and Lamberts Colladeen (£12.95).

how long do I have to use it before I get any results?

Lots of our testers asked this, and with cellulite products it really depends what results you are expecting. Many of those that came out top in our survey gave instant results – and by that we don't mean they got rid of our tester's cellulite overnight, but made a marked difference to the look of their skin. Which makes a big difference to the overall picture. We think you should follow the usage guidelines (products worth buying have clear ones) until you have used all of the product. Then take a view.

'work up a sweat: as well as exercising, soaking in a warm bath (after exfoliating your entire body) with a sprinkling of Epsom or mineral salts in it will encourage your body to sweat and cleanse itself naturally'

shopping for cellulite products

Before you head for the shops or flash your cash:

1. Have a little talk with yourself and agree that you won't be swayed by anti-cellulite products which claim to get rid of your cellulite. Wake up and smell the coffee: no product is going to get rid of your saddlebags or flabby tum. Repeat after us: I will not be taken in, I will not...
2. Take a close look at the ingredients: the main (and often most potent) ones in these treatments are those which have a draining effect on the fluid that is held in the upper layers of your skin, and which clarify skin, stimulate and tone it. So look for essential oils such as juniper, rosemary, cypress and geranium, plus caffeine, horsetail, butcher's broom and seabroom (a form of brown seaweed which also appears on the labelling as halopteris scoparia).
3. Decide how much you want to spend: we know that you are prepared to invest in expensive products if they are effective – which is just as well because the results of our tests showed that the more expensive body contourers or cellulite products *did* work best. So if cellulite bothers you enough and you are serious about tackling it (i.e. you are going to follow a diet and exercise plan) it might be worth spending that bit more for peace of mind.

... cellulite products we rate:

Julia Shiseido Body Creator Lotion (£29.95 for 200ml): 'I love this for its fragrance, fast absorption and the fact that it takes no effort to apply. It hasn't got rid of my cellulite but it's definitely improved things.'

Kate Leirac Sensorielle Drainage Cream (£19.95 for 200ml): 'Of all the contouring products I've tried, nothing touches this in terms of performance as far as I'm concerned. It takes down fluid retention and in doing so noticeably streamlines areas prone to puff. It's French, and the French understand problems like this better than anyone else in the world. Mayaltha Better Cycles (£20.95 for 175ml) – a diuretic serum which you put on your abdomen, thighs and arms; and Malki Dead Sea Salts (£6.99 for 1kg) – which you bath in – great at easing pre-menstrual bloating which makes cellulite look worse.'

the 9 best cellulite products

the mission To find you the most effective and user-friendly cellulite treatments on the market.

the criteria *At no point did we ask our testers to start measuring their thighs*. They judged the cellulite products they tried on their ability to better the look of the overlying skin by improving local circulation, drainage and tone; making it firmer, smoother, softer and less puffy, dry and goosepimply. We feel that if this is effective enough it can offset the appearance of cellulite to a point where you won't care whether you have got it or not, which is the healthiest attitude. A real decider was the scent (many of our testers said they would not use a product if it didn't have a passable smell – even if it worked well), and the product's instructions; some of the people who responded to our survey said that on many products they are not clear enough.

Guerlain Issima Body Secret Ice Lift Treatment

£35 for 200ml

'No promises to get rid of cellulite – which works in its favour as far as I'm concerned,' said Catherine (48), one of the people who gave this product full marks. 'Its main aim is to lift your skin – something that I never thought would help my thigh problem – I always thought in inches. But it definitely makes my legs look better.' A winning feature is the instant icy sensation it gives when you put it on – all part of the lifting and toning effect: 'It cools instantly, perking up hot tired legs,' said Julianna (60). She was so impressed by the scent she wrote, 'It makes you feel like you have been to a beautiful spa and swum in Alpine waters.'

the science bit: This has got all the big drainage and stimulating ingredients in it – gingko biloba, coleus and caffeine, plus Guerlain's potent nourishing complex Blue Gold (a blend of pure gold and and abyssal algae); the 'icy thrill' effect is generated by the product's texture and mentholated scent.

Spiezia Anti Cellulite Oil

£19.20 for 100ml

'If you ask me, this is what the ideal anti-cellulite product should be,' remarked Carina (31). 'For a start it's an oil – something professional masseurs use; second it's organic – and if you're following an anti-cellulite diet and trying to cut down on toxic food like coffee that makes sense; and lastly it really does help to get rid of fluid retention – my big problem.' This product is also highly rated because being an oil it facilitates that all-important massage applicatory action – something many creams don't do because they evaporate or disappear into your skin too quickly.

the science bit: A blend of potent organic oils – jojoba, wheatgerm, olive, sesame and wheatgerm – plus stimulating rosemary essential oil.

Thalgo Thalgomince Massage Cream

£26.50 for 150ml

Philly (32) was one of the testers who said she thought this product deserved full marks for effort. 'I've had the FrigiThalgo wrap treatment in the past,' she said, 'and it was really, really good, so I wondered whether the cream would work as well. And it *is* great – maybe because it's French? It takes a while to rub it in but that's the whole point – you have to do the massage to improve the cellulite areas. I would buy it because I can't afford regular massage and this is a great DIY version.'

the science bit: The magic ingredients are firming horsetail extract and Thalgo's special phyto-refining complex which they claim breaks down fat.

Phytomer Bodydelic Unique Anti-Cellulite Cream

£23 for 150ml

Bridget (38) said, 'I've got the softest, smoothest skin I've ever had – the bumpy bits are still there, but my stomach and thighs still look acceptable – something must be working.' Laura (35) thinks there is a 'general smoothing difference' on the backs of her thighs and said, 'I'm persevering with it because I think it might be having an effect on my cellulite. But it has definitely made my skin softer and more supple which does improve things anyway.'

the science bit: A plant ingredient called seabroom – which Phytomer say stops fat cells from forming and increases production of collagen (the stuff that makes skin elastic and supple) – is the key to this formula. Being an oil-in-water-in-oil emulsion encourages it to absorb into skin quickly.

Aromatherapy Associates Detox Cellulite Gel

£20 for 200ml

Despite the dreaded 'detox' word, this gel converted several cynics among our testers. Annie (39) wrote, 'I can't believe how easy and painless it's been to deal with my cellulite. I thought I'd worry about it forever, but having made an effort – which to be honest wasn't that much of one – to massage this into my legs every night before I got into bed, I feel 100 per cent more confident about my figure. It's really bizarre. The lumps and bumps are still there, but my legs are definitely firmer, and my skin is brighter and clearer.' Our testers also liked the gel's cooling effects and one admitted she keeps it in the fridge to 'increase the sensation'.

the science bit: This is a potent mix of really good quality draining and stimulating aromatherapy oils – juniper, grape, pine and rosemary.

Leirac Sensorielle Drainage Cream

£19.95 for 200ml

'Kate is always banging on about this cream and how marvellous it is so I wanted to see if it worked for me,' said Sarah (42). 'The big test was my jeans: if I could do the zip up without a struggle at the height of my PMT – when I get bad water retention and my cellulite looks much worse – I'd give it the thumbs up. Not only did it make a huge difference to my water retention and stop me feeling all puffy, but it made my skin warm and supple too. I didn't think products like this existed.'

the science bit: There are two groups of active ingredients in this cream – draining plant extracts like gingko biloba, elder and butcher's broom, and cyclatella, an ingredient which stimulates the natural endorphins and hormones under the surface of your skin where much of fluid retention occurs.

Caudalie Draining & Relaxing Bath Oil

£27 for 125ml

Lots of beauty companies and aromatherapists have developed 'detoxifying' bath oils, but few of them do much more than make your bath smell nice. This bath oil, developed at the Caudalie spa in France, was the most effective of all those tested. 'It's like a cross between an oil and a gel,' said Margaret (62). 'You just put five drops to your bath when you are feeling a bit bloated and it really seems to take the puffiness down. It hasn't got rid of my cellulite, but it definitely makes my thighs and calves feel much less puffy, tight and heavy – which to me is half the battle.'

the science bit: As well as red vine extract, which has a strengthening effect on blood capillaries and improves circulation, it contains juniper berry oil – which has a draining effect – and purifying cypress oil, geranium and lavender.

Clarins Anti-Eau Body Oil

£27.50 for 100ml

One of Clarins all-time heroes and although it doesn't strictly say it works on cellulite it certainly helps to improve matters. Shirley (50) wrote: 'Everything about this product is superb: it smells wonderful, it works very well – a definite draining action – and it warms up your skin which is a first for me because my thighs are always cold; it absorbs well and is easy to use. No complaints; it meets the criteria.'

the science bit: A potent blend of essential oils broom, geranium and marjoram in hazelnut oil which have a deep-cleansing, stimulating and toning effect.

Mayaltha Better Bottom

£20.75 for 175ml

Kate really rates the Australian Mayaltha body system and this was the only product in the range she had not tried so she asked Lizzie (47) to road test it for us. 'When I first saw it I thought they were having me on,' Lizzie said. 'And I thought if it does anything for my bum it *will* be a miracle product. It's still big and lumpy. But this product – a sort of cold jelly – makes it noticeably tighter and firmer; it's like putting on a pair of support tights, a bit bizarre. Packaging gets the thumbs up too: there is lots of blurb about the ingredients and how to use the product inside the box.'

the science bit: As well as horse chestnut and witch hazel (which have an astringent action on blood capillaries), natural exfoliators citric, lactic and glycolic acid and wild fennel essential oil (a diuretic), this serum contains cyclodextrin, said to strengthen collagen – the stuff that makes skin firm.

hair removal

For most of us, de-fuzzing our bodies is a daily necessity. Others don't see a bit of underarm hair as a big deal – as long as it's only a bit. As a nation we are not keen on 'excess' hair (by which we mean hair that is anywhere but on your head), and buy hair removers and depilatories as habitually as hygiene staples like toothpaste.

We also all seem to be on an eternal search for a better hair remover (and mascara). This has a lot to do with marketing. Beauty companies go to the most extraordinary lengths to make hair removal sexy, naming girlie-pink razors after goddesses and giving them extra duties (like moisturising skin) other than shaving. At the end of the day though, hair removal is hair removal. It's as boring as that. And hair removers and depilatories (two different things – we'll explain all in a minute) can't do much more than this, despite some of the amazing claims they make.

'don't shave or wax just after exfoliating or before going in the sun – it hurts'

So it's pretty simple then: what you want is a hair remover which does the job – of whipping off (or out) the offenders – effectively and with the least amount of fuss. And two or three of our testers said they wanted the hair-free results to last longer, too.

This is where we come in. The first beauty column we wrote together for *The Daily Mail* a few years ago was on hair removal: we were despatched to try as many products as possible and report back on their performances. And having worked our way through at least a dozen hair removers each for the benefit of *Daily Mail* readers – and setting fire to one of our kitchens in the process (don't ask) – you could say that we have done our homework on this subject.

There is nothing we don't know about hair removal (even though neither of us are especially hairy), so rest assured that the products which have made the grade for this particular section of the book are the best your money can buy. By the way, there are various products which claim to retard or

do you really have to do a patch test before using a new depilatory?

Yes. It's as boring as priming walls for paint but there is logic behind it: depilatories contain very strong ingredients which 'dissolve' hair and they can irritate – it makes sense when you think that hair and skin are very similar in make-up, so chemicals that destroy hair can also destroy skin. Test on a tiny patch on the inside of your forearm.

inhibit hair growth. We can't see how a topical product could ever honour this claim, but perhaps you could let us know if it worked for you?

depilatories v hair removers

What is the difference and is either more effective than the other?

depilatories These are creams which literally melt hair away and they can be very effective, but they don't always agree with everyone because the ingredients – usually calcium hydroxide and sodium or calcium thioglycolate – are quite aggressive. As well as removing your unwanted hair some depilatories claim to retard regrowth and make your hairs grow back finer and lighter than before, but this is nonsense: hairs may reappear faster after removing hair by *shaving* (because you only whip off the hair not the root) but your genes and hormones are the only factors that can determine hair growth and texture.

you get the best results from depilatories if you warm your skin up first (we suggest de-fuzzing after a bath or shower) because it softens the hairs and encourages your pores to 'let go' of them more easily.

hair removers Waxes, sugars and razors remove hairs *without* the help of chemicals. We won't beat about the bush on this, waxing and sugaring are a total pfaff – even if you don't have to heat or mix anything up, it's so much easier (and less painful) to shave in the bath. But although easy – and the hair removal method most women fall back on for legs and bikini line – shaving provides the least satisfactory results. Hairs pop out faster because you only nick off the hair – the root stays put, so you get stubble and sometimes red bumps. Waxes and sugars, on the other hand, do tend to have longer-lasting results than shaving because they rip the hair (plus root) out from below the top layer of your skin rather than just skimming it off on the surface.

you get the best results from waxes and sugars if you apply the products in the direction of hair growth. This means once hairs are embedded in the wax or sugar mix pull it all off *in the direction of hair growth* and the hairs come out more easily.

you get the best results from shaving if you use a proper shaving mousse or oil (instead of soap) with your razor – on wet skin – and apply unscented moisturiser to your skin afterwards to reduce irritation. Don't exfoliate before removing hair – it can over-sensitise your skin; a much gentler way to shift dry bits of skin is to add a pinch of baking soda to your shaving mousse. The best way to get rid of red bumps is to dissolve a couple of asprin (it has good anti-inflammatory properties) in half a glass of cold water and dab the solution onto your skin with cottonwool.

shopping for depilatories & hair removers

Before you head for the shops or flash your cash:

1. Consider whether you want a depilatory or hair remover – there is a difference in technique and time.
2. If possible, smell depilatories. If it isn't possible, stick to our guide to weed out depilatories that have an acceptable smell – their 'scent' is very important because, as you told us when we did our survey, no matter how good a product is, if it smells revolting you won't use it.
3. Decide how much you want to spend – our road test proved that you can pick up a decent depilatory or hair remover for around a fiver.

... hair removers we rate:

Julia Gillette For Women Venus (£5.59): 'I'm a razor girl. I can't be doing with home waxing or creams, too messy and too smelly.'

Kate 'Ditto. I can't see how much simpler you can make hair removal.'

the 4 best depilatories & hair removers

the mission To find you the most effective and user-friendly depilatories and hair removers on the market.

the criteria Our testers judged the depilatories and hair removers they tried on their efficacy, speed, performance, smell, instructions (our testers said that these are often not clear) and longevity – you want the results to last, yes, but lots of you also want the product to last longer than a few weeks, too.

Nads Hair Removal £18.95 for 6oz

Melissa (17) isn't particularly hairy but was dying to try this for us because she had read so much about it. And her verdict was one of the most positive: 'It's so easy to use,' she said. 'You don't even need to heat it up because it works best at room temperature. You just spread the gel over your skin (I did my legs) press a cloth strip on top and pull it off. It pulls all your hairs out, not just the longest ones as some hair removers do, and the pain wasn't so bad. I'm so glad I tried it.'

the science bit: NADS is one of the very few beauty products which is totally natural: you can eat it which is a good litmus test for any product which claims to be natural – it is made from honey, molasses, lemon juice and vinegar.

Body Shop Sugaring

£6.50 for 200ml, spatula £1, strips £2.50

'Testing this filled me with horror,' admitted Mary-Ann (39). 'I thought I was really doing "you two" a big favour because the thought of putting something sugary all over my legs instead of the usual few swipes with a razor was awful. But I was really surprised. It's not sticky (my biggest fear), it's incredibly easy to use and it works very well – so well in fact that I've used it twice since first trying it and I reckon I'll get at least a dozen more applications out of it. Good price too.'

the science bit: The formula is simple – sugar, water and sandalwood oil, which has a smoothing and calming effect on your skin.

Veet Mousse (originally Immac)

£5.25 for 200ml

To be honest, we were hoping to come up with a surprise winner in this category – not the usual contender. But our testers unanimously gave this product top marks, so there was no getting around it. Sarah (44) and Juliet (36) both tried it for the first time and said they would buy it again because it worked so well. 'I thought it would smell,' said Juliet, 'because I remember my sister using it years ago and it stank the house out. That's why I've never used it myself. But they've obviously done something to it because it doesn't smell bad now and I can't fault its performance: hair-free legs in no time.' Sarah's only gripe is that you get through it very quickly.

the science bit: The key ingredient is potassium thioglycolate, which weakens and dissolves the hairs. It also contains vitamin E and soothing aloe vera. And you can use this spray-on mousse on your legs, underarms and bikini line.

Hair Solutions Advanced Wax Strips

£4.95 for 16 single-sided strips (which, if you are desperate, can be re-used)

Trudie (42) was one of four testers who gave these the thumbs up – even though she normally uses a depilatory cream. 'I've been looking for an excuse to try hair-waxing strips,' she said, 'and I'm glad I did! There are clear usage instructions on the packet – even though the strips are foolproof – and I really like this method. The strips work amazingly well even though all you have to do is rub them between your hands to warm them, stick them on your skin for a minute and rip them off.'

the science bit: The strips are impregnated with antiseptic tea tree oil, and you also get a soothing post-wax lotion containing tea tree oil, lavender and lemon.

HAIR CARE

Don't tell us – *we know*: hair care – the huge market that is shampoo, conditioner and styling products – is an absolute minefield. How anyone ever manages to find their way around the rows and rows of products is a mystery even to us and we are the experts!

While much of the hairdressing fraternity see hair (and hair styling) as an 'art form', most of us just want the right shampoo and conditioner for our hair and perhaps the odd styling product. If only it were this simple. Unfortunately, the size and changeability of the market makes it very tricky to find those products. In fact most of our testers admitted to being baffled and disillusioned by hair care.

You said you rarely bought the same product twice; and that you spent your lives trying new products that promised the world but supplied very little. You are more likely to buy products with names that tell you what they do – i.e. BIG HAIR; you find products with names as long as a sentence – a habit peculiar to hair care – a complete turn-off (are you listening hair companies?), and often feel that companies try to blind you with science. As one tester put it, 'Do they think we will buy a shampoo if it sounds more scientific?'

Both of us have worked with hairstylists in one way or another throughout our careers and noticed that they only ever have one or two key products in their kitbags. So why are the rest of us presented with thousands of different options, half of which seem to be superfluous to our needs?

Make no mistake, the hair care business is about big bucks and (it must be said) even bigger egos. And that applies as much to the giant hair care conglomerates as the independent salons and stylists. The hair care market is based on hype and image; and the only way to avoid ending up with products that only look good on your bathroom shelf is to refuse to be swayed by the marketing.

Or get some good objective advice.

What you will find out about in this chapter:

- That you don't need to spend more than £20 on shampoo
- Why 'two-in-ones' (shampoo-conditioners) don't go
- Whether grey hair needs special shampoo
- That the best shampoos for scaly scalps are not necessarily coal-tar based
- That conditioner can stretch out the time between highlighting sessions
- Which products stop your hair going frizzy when it rains

shampoo

What makes you buy a shampoo? The bottle? Its claims for bigger/thicker/shinier hair? Or the fact that the person behind the formula is a famous hairdresser?

At the end of the day what most of us want is a shampoo that cleans our hair and injects some volume into it if needed. If it brightens up highlights that have been dulled by hard water, straightens out frizz or makes our hair look more polished, too – that is a bonus.

> 'don't waste your money on 'anti-build-up' shampoos: just swap around a couple of shampoos with each wash'

We are not very loyal though (why should we be with so much choice?): if a new shampoo arrives on the shelves with enough hype we will give it a try, especially if it claims to do something really revolutionary like wash our hair and condition it at the same time.

The responses we got to our survey told us that many of you chop and change hair care products constantly because you allow yourselves to be led by hype, you are confused about what your hair actually needs (again, because of conflicting hype) and you aren't even sure how many products you should be using at any given time.

Hair care is a massive business, and shampoos – along with styling products – are perhaps the most fickle side of it. Just as we pick and choose shampoos, rarely coming back to the same one, shampoo trends come and go as manufacturers dress-up the same basic formulas to give hair more body, shine or curl depending on fashion.

Read on to find out which ones perform most successfully.

what makes a good shampoo?

1. **One that makes cleaning its main priority:** many make a big deal about extra bonuses like re-moisturising your hair or brightening up your highlights, and lots of our testers said they love shampoos that do more than one job because they feel they are getting value for money. The most important thing though is to get a shampoo that *cleans your hair and scalp properly*; if it manages to make your hair look fuller, or your highlights brighter, that is a bonus.
2. **One that doesn't have an off-putting smell:** there is nothing worse than walking around all day with your head in a cloud of synthetic fragrance.
3. **One that doesn't strip your hair** and leave it dry like straw, no matter how hard the water is in your house.

is baby shampoo better for your hair?

A lot of women ask us this – usually those who like to wash their hair everyday and feel that their shampoo should be mild. But baby shampoo doesn't necessarily clean your hair as well as adult shampoo because its key cleansing ingredient isn't strong enough. It's fine for babies and children who don't use conditioner or styling products, but not necessarily for you: buy your own!

clearing up some grey areas

By the age of 50 at least half of us have got grey (colourless) hair. Why it happens is still largely a mystery. What scientists do know is that hair goes grey when melanocytes in the bulb stop making the pigment they put into hair as it grows. But no one really knows why this happens; and the race is now on to develop a really effective hair care product (and it could be a shampoo) that will make the pigment-making process active again and permanently restore the pigment to colourless hair. This is something many of our testers told us would be their dream hair care product, along with a hair 'mascara' that temporarily painted out grey and covers up roots.

The breakthrough is getting closer and closer, but in the meantime, does grey hair need special care? Well, it tends to be a bit wirier – so it could be drier, and if this is the case you may benefit from a more moisturising shampoo or conditioner. And if your hair is 100 percent grey, it can be quite dull-looking; your shampoo should clarify it so it looks brighter. On the whole though we don't think shampoos specially formulated for grey hair are worth buying – especially if they are expensive.

shopping for shampoos

Before you head for the shops or flash your cash:

1. **Decide what kind of shampoo you want:** one which cleanses and volumises or straightens frizz, moisturises your hair, enhances its colour or revives your highlights. It helps to narrow the choice down. Knowing whether you have hard or soft water can also help when it comes to choosing shampoo. Some contain ingredients that counteract the effects of hard water – which dries out your hair and scalp. Lush – whose hard water shampoo came out best in our road test – did a survey recently to find out where the best (and worst) places in the UK are for washing your hair. They found that Edinburgh is the best (lots of lovely soft water there) and Basingstoke is the worst.
2. **Decide how much you want to spend:** our testers found that competitively-priced shampoos performed as well as mid- and top-range ones (even better in some cases), which adds more weight to our belief that there is no gain in spending a lot of money on shampoo – certainly not more than £15 or £20 anyway. Expensive shampoo is purely a marketing exercise, and one that doesn't deserve to succeed in our view.

why two-in-ones don't go

Ask any hairdresser and they will tell you to use separate shampoo and conditioner – not a shampoo which claims to do both. Why? 'Because although they make your hair feel soft and look shiny to begin with, two-in-one shampoos contain silicates that coat your hair and ultimately sap its lustre,' says Michaeljohn's Michael Rasser. So there you go – finally, a simple answer to a question many of our testers asked.

... shampoos we rate:

Julia Dermalogica Shine Therapy Shampoo (£13.50 for 237ml): 'This is a long-time favourite of mine. It smells wonderful and fresh and gives my hair – which is chemically-treated – some life and shine.'

Kate Kerastase Bain Volumactiv (£8.80 for 250ml): 'Another discovery I made early on in my beauty writing career that hasn't yet been toppled from my all-time fave list. It makes your hair feel so full of air and volume it swings like a kilt.'

the 9 best shampoos

the mission to find you the most effective and user-friendly shampoos on the market.

the criteria our testers judged the shampoos they tried on their ability to clean their hair and in doing so, enhance its shine, colour and softness. They also tested shampoos on their smell, the effect they had on their hair afterwards – whether they made it bouncy or lank – the impact they had on their scalps, and whether they were good value for money.

Nexxus Y Serum Shampoo For Younger Looking Hair

£5.90 for 150ml

The name of this shampoo is a bit dodgy – *shampoo for younger-looking hair?* Sounds a bit too much like marketing flannel to us, and yet it proved to be such a popular shampoo – every single one of our testers loved it so much they clearly overlooked its other ambitions. Liz (64) tried it – and its complementary conditioner – and thought both 'excellent'. Linda (44) gave it a 10/10 and commented: 'It made my hair bouncy, shiny and thick-looking. A friend of mine even asked me if I'd had my highlights redone because my hair looked revitalised. It must be good.' And Candice (21) made an interesting remark: 'It's best for Afro hair – in fact a lot of Afro hairdressers recommend it even though it's not marketed as such.'

the science bit: key ingredients are Y Serum, an 'anti-ageing' complex of green tea and yamabushitake mushroom. These are antioxidants also put in anti-ageing creams, and the aim is to revive hair which has become coarse, dry and dull with age.

Black Like Me Protein Moisturising Shampoo

£2.99 for 250ml

Afro hair needs lots of extra moisture – especially when it has been chemically treated – as it loses it very easily. This South African range is made specifically for Afro hair, but some products in the range also work well on naturally curly and colour-treated hair. Angie (31), who has straightened Afro hair, tried this shampoo for us and said, 'My hair is obviously drier than it should be but this shampoo treats it more kindly than most. I left it on for a few minutes as recommended and it made it much softer. I'd use it again for sure.'

the science bit: the formula includes wheat germ proteins that improve condition (without making hair lank), and that strengthen and protect hair.

Redken All Soft Shampoo

£8 for 300ml

This shampoo has got a reputation for reviving hair which is frazzled (exposure to sun, sea and wind, over-styling with sticky products, too much heat-styling, etc.) and in need of a bit of TLC. It also cuts down on frizz – a problem for lots of the people who took part in our survey. We didn't ask Kate (42) what she had been up to with her hair, but she was one of the testers who was very keen on this shampoo, saying it brought her dry hair back to life. 'I give this a 10/10, it's really excellent,' she wrote. 'It actually detangled and softened my hair and it looks amazingly healthy.'

the science bit: the key ingredients are avocado oil which claims to restore moisture by trapping it in the hair, and moisturising glycerine. The formula works to iron-out frizz by softening and flattening the cuticles on each strand.

Kerastase Dermo-Calm Shampoo

£8.80 for 250ml

We think this is the first shampoo which actually addresses the problem of 'flakiness', a sensitive or stressed scalp, without making the problem worse. That might sound a bit controversial, but have you tried those shampoos which claim to shift dandruff yet leave you with a scalp that feels like it has been stretched over your head like an elastic band? 'Soft, creamy and it left my scalp calm, clean and without build-up which makes it dirty again within a day. My hair is shiny and smooth,' is how Leah (55) describes its effects. Stress is one of the main causes of an itchy, crusty (we're not afraid of that word – 'flakiness' is not the same thing – come on hair care companies!) scalp – as Simon (37) knows: 'When I'm tired, tense and stressed I scratch my head – it's probably a nerve thing,' he said. 'I felt this shampoo calmed my scalp down considerably, at least making it more comfortable.'

the science bit: includes a Hydra-Destress Complex which is made up of sunflower oil and an ingredient called calophyllum which both calm irritation, plus piroctone olamine – an anti-dandruff property – and moisturising glycerine. There are two variants – one for dry and one for normal/combination hair.

Pantene Pro-V Clarifying Shampoo

£1.99 for 200ml

This no-fuss, basic shampoo met all our testing criteria and came out as the best all-round hair cleanser; it shifts dirt and grease, and works well as a mild substitute when you want to swap around shampoos to prevent build-up. It is decently priced too, so good value for money. Our testers said it left their hair looking clean, healthy and shiny. 'Just one wash was enough. For three days my hair looked and felt great. I'm glad I've got over any preconceived ideas about the cheaper brand shampoos not being as good,' said Isabel (27). 'I've obviously been spending more than I need to.'

the science bit: contains surfactants like laureth sulphate which lift dirt and product residue off hair and scalp, a pH balancer called sodium citrate and very little conditioning properties – which is why it looks crystal clear.

Charles Worthington Dream Hair Heavenly Hairwash Outrageously Rich Shampoo

£4.99 for 250ml

Everything about this shampoo – from its packaging to its fragrance – is supposed to make you think 'luxury'; yet it is economical because you only need to do one wash to get the best results. Helena (28) has long hair that she works hard to keep in top condition: 'I go back to this shampoo simply because my hair always looks better when I use it,' she said. 'The shampoo lathers up well, it has a lovely fragrance and it doesn't make my hair all knotty.'

the science bit: contains a Damage Deflector which sounds like something out of Thunderbirds but it is an antioxidising blend of green tea extracts.

Redken Fresh Curls Shampoo

£8 for 300ml

'Love it, love it, love it. Great smell and lovely to use,' said Melanie (42), who we think possibly loved it. In fact, this was the only shampoo for non-Afro curly hair that came out with completely positive results, and Melanie – who has very long curly and gorgeous hair – was the perfect guineau pig. It gives curls definition – so they don't just fall flat – control and lots of moisture (curly hair is often drier than straight). Sophie (23), who has a shorter mop of curls, said: 'This is such a good product. I wish it was cheaper, but as it has made my hair so much easier to control I think I would spend that amount on it anyway.'

the science bit: ingredients include natural honey to moisturise, calcium to stabilise the shape of the curl and coconut oil to soften, smooth and add shine.

Aveda Colour Enhancer Shampoo

£7.50 for 250ml

Many shampoos claim to enhance or preserve hair colour and highlights, but to be honest it was really difficult to find one which made a noticeable difference. Our testers thought the products they tried were 'okay' and 'nice to use', but nothing stood out as being exceptional except this range. Caroline (23) tried one of the shampoos and gave it the thumbs up for its 'wonderful, fresh fragrance', and Genevieve (35) gave the shampoos 10/10 because she said they are 'always reliable and smell great'. Camomile for blonde and lighter shades of hair was very popular: Dierdre (38) said, 'It made a noticeable difference to the brightness of my hair,' and another well-liked shampoo in the range turned out to be Black Malva for darker hair. 'My hair is very long and I colour it because I'm so grey. This is the only shampoo I've used that keeps its colour true and glossy,' said Claire (42).

the science bit: uses organically grown camomile to enhance light coloured hair, or black malva, a flowering herb known for its emollient properties.

Lush Hard £3.90 for 100gm (cut straight from the block in the shop)

Lush are a truly innovative beauty company. They manage to make products which are fun to use but have a genuinely practical quality, and this shampoo is a good example of that. Although Sarah-Jane (39) doesn't live in Basingstoke – the city identified by Lush as having the hardest water in the UK – she does have hard water. She wasn't sure about using a solid shampoo but was impressed by the way this one counteracted the effects of hard water. 'It took a few washes for my hair to feel softer,' she said. 'But my scalp was less flaky from the start and you can tell it's different to regular shampoos right away because you don't have to use much of it – so it's great value – and it lathers up easily. I have to use a lot of shampoo normally just to get a lather. If you don't get a lather your hair doesn't feel so clean. I'll definitely keep buying this.'

the science bit: the key ingredients are sesqui carbonate, a natural water softener, soy lecithin and eggs, which fortify and soften hair.

conditioners

It's amazing to think that there was a time when conditioner didn't even exist; but the fact that it does is actually testament to the effectiveness of modern shampoos.

Before the Second World War, shampoo didn't clean hair as well as it does now, and people had to use vinegar or lemon as a rinse to get the residue off and make their hair look clean and shiny. Now of course it is all more involved, and few of us would – or could – dream of washing our hair without conditioning afterwards.

> 'the only cure for split ends is scissors. But adding a bit of scrum to the ends can stop them from sticking out'

Conditioners finish the job. They should make your hair more manageable, smoother, softer and shinier. They are made of emollients that flatten cuticles on the strands – which makes hair look shinier because it allows light to reflect off the surface more evenly – and should soften and detangle hair without weighing it down.

Conditioners also help cut down on static and protect hair from being damaged by ultraviolet (UV) rays. But despite some promises to mend split ends (made, we assume, because this is a common problem – in fact lots of our testers said that if such a product existed they would buy it), that job belongs to your hairdresser's scissors.

So which ones are the best? Read on to find out.

what makes a good conditioner?

1. **Smell** – *so* important, especially if it's a leave-in one: there is nothing worse than the smell of conditioner lingering over you all day long, and – as ever – many of our testers said that however good a product is, they won't use it if they don't like the way it smells.
2. **Texture** – if a conditioner is too thick and creamy it can make your hair greasy again within a couple of days (less if it's a leave-in one); if it's too watery it won't perform properly. Choose a texture somewhere inbetween.
3. **One that can be used sparingly** – some lightweight conditioners make you feel as if you have to apply masses to get results; the best ones dispense the right amount.

how often should you use conditioner?

You can condition too much. In fact, one of the main reasons for dull, lank hair – and short lifespans of perms and other chemical treatments – is over-conditioning. So how much is too much? Well, you only really need to condition after every wash (and for many of us this means everyday) if your hair is naturally curly or frizzy, or very dry. Most hair only needs conditioner on the ends because hair closer to the scalp is naturally protected by the skin's own secretions.

how to use conditioner

1. Towel-dry your hair after washing it.
2. Apply a coin-sized drop of conditioner to your hands like cream and massage it into the ends of your hair. Very few people need to apply conditioner from roots to tips – only those with very dry hair – and applying it to the ends is more economical, especially if it's a leave-in conditioner.
3. Comb your hair through very gently – it loses about a quarter of its elasticity when it's wet and if you tug you will break it. If it's long, hold it as you comb so you don't put too much pressure on the roots; a wide-toothed comb is perfect for this job.
4. After a minute rinse it out thoroughly (until the water runs completely clean and bubble-free) with hot water. Then give it a final rinse of cold water to flatten the cuticles and boost shine.

how long should you leave conditioner on your hair?

It depends what kind of conditioner you use. Most conditioners only coat your hair – they are not absorbed by the strands – so they are as effective after only one minute as they are after ten. Oil or panthenol-based conditioners – usually deep treatments or hair masks – do penetrate the hair shaft and so they should be left on for longer.

... conditioners we rate:

Julia Dermalogica Silk Finish Conditioner (£16.60 for 237ml): 'It's the perfect partner to the Dermalogica shampoo I use. It's light, so I don't feel like I'm overloading my hair – which is easy to do because there are so many unnecessary products.'

Kate Michaeljohn SalonSpa Super Detangling Leave-In Conditioner (£4.99 for 150ml): 'If I didn't use conditioner I'd be combing my hair out all day after washing it. This product does the work for you – it's amazing – and makes your hair feel like silk.'

the 6 best conditioners

the mission: to find you the most effective and user-friendly conditioners on the market.

the criteria our testers judged the conditioners they tried on their ability to soften, moisturise and detangle their hair, as well as enhance its shine. They also tested conditioners for their smell and the effect they had on their scalp and hair afterwards – whether they made the strands bouncy or limp, and whether they considered them to be good value for money.

Aussie 3 Minute Miracle Conditioner £5.29 for 250ml

This Australian range was popular with our testers generally. Lots of them said they would buy the products again and again because they know they work really well – reason enough to make our best list. Several of our testers commented specifically on this conditioner: 'I've been using it for years and have never felt the need to look for another conditioner because it works a treat,' wrote Zoe (27). It can be used on a daily basis if you need it, but doesn't make hair lifeless or weigh it down as many do when you use them a lot – although we would recommend only applying it to the ends.

the science bit: uses extracts of Australian Balm Mint to smooth cuticles and repair damaged hair, and aims to inject body and shine into hair.

Michaeljohn SalonSpa Super Detangling Leave-In Conditioner

£4.99 for 150ml

Loved by Kate and many of our testers because it is so easy to use – a leave-in detangling and conditioning spray which kicks hair back into shape after the day-to-day abuse it gets. Like lots of us with long thick hair, Anneka (28) admits she hates combing her hair after washing it. 'It's usually one big mass of mess!' she remarked. 'This made life so much easier though. I didn't wince once when combing it through and my hair looks fab.' It also seems to keep frizz to a minimum – something it is often assumed that people with straight hair don't have a problem with. But as some of our testers confirm, they do.

the science bit: the key ingredients are avocado and sweet almond oils which help hair detangle more easily. It is also full of wonderful aromatherapy essences like lavender, patchouli, juniper berry and camomile.

Kerastase Lait Après-Soleil Cheveux Naturels/Colorés

£11.50 for 150ml

From the answers we got in our survey not many of you bother to change your hair care products or protect your hair when you are on holiday, even though you know that the sun gives it a rough time. However, some of our testers agreed to take some holiday hair care products away with them to try and this conditioner got their best vote. 'It made my sun-singed mop much more manageable and less straw-like,' said Victoria (37). 'It really improved the shine and condition.' Nicky (27) – who admits she doesn't give her hair much attention at home either or spend much money on hair care products – remarked that, 'It is expensive but I think it's worth it. My hair hasn't looked this good or felt so soft for ages.'

the science bit: developed to maintain coloured and natural hair when you are in the sun, the formula includes ceramides which fortify the strands' natural protective barrier, and pro-vitamin B5, which repairs dry and damaged hair.

Big Sexy Hair Big Volume Conditioner

£5.60 for 250ml

Yes, we are talking BIG here: big bottle, big letters on the bottle and big results. The conditioner is also quick and easy to use – you just apply it, concentrating on the ends of your hair, and rinse out without waiting. It moisturises hair without weighing it down – key, because this conditioner promises to condition and volumise. 'Never used this range before and I thought I'd tried every volumising product there is,' said the once limp-haired Sophie (31). 'It really lifted my hair – right from the root – and when I blow-dried it the results were spectacular: seriously volumised hair!'

the science bit: includes pro-vitamin B5 to repair hair and smooth frizz, as well as wholewheat proteins (the magic volumisers) and panthenol which adds shine.

Nicky Clarke Hairomatherapy Colour Care 60 Second Secret Intensive Treatment

£6.49 for 150ml

If you have got all the time in the world to sit in the bath with a lovely hair mask on this isn't the product for you. Most of us don't have the luxury of time – life just isn't like that – which is why Nicky has developed a deep-working conditioner that claims to work extra speedily. And the product proved to be a hit with our testers. 'A great fragrance to it, but best of all, it makes my limp hair look FANTASTIC and zaps static,' said Deborah (33). Sophie (19) said, 'I need to wash my hair everyday and always use conditioner. This is quick-working and can be relied on to do the same thing – make my hair soft and shiny.' Our testers are a beady-eyed bunch and several commented on the product's new-ish packaging, asking 'Why did it had to be changed, we liked the old style?' Um ..

the science bit: uses essences of ylang ylang and sandalwood to give hair protection whilst protecting and healing as well

Trevor Sorbie Body & Bounce Fine Hair Leave-In Conditioner

£3.99 for 250ml

So you don't bother with conditioner (especially a leave-in one) because you have got fine hair and think it will make it limper? No longer a problem thanks to clever Trevor, who noticed a demand for a lightweight conditioner that would soften fine hair (which often becomes coarser and drier with age), enhance its volume, condition and shine. So he developed a spray-on one. 'My hair is so thin but I still have difficulty taming it,' wrote Michelle (32). 'I tried this conditioner and found it gave my hair more body and enabled me to style it properly – without it going all over the place.'

the science bit: contains panthenol to replenish moisture, and an ingredient called polyquarternium 10, a conditioning film-forming polymer which smoothes down cuticles and injects body into hair.

the top 3 deep-conditioning hair treatments

Daniel Galvin Miracle Solution Colour Shine Brightener

£4.99 for Shine Brightener Powder (7gms), Shine Brightener Lotion (93ml) and Finishing Conditioning Treatment (10ml)

For all those people who did our survey and said that their dream hair care product would be one that significantly 'revived their colour or highlights', this is a product worth trying. Somehow it is not just the roots that make it look depressed; hair that needs a colour boost often looks dull and flat too – it needs an injection of life. This one-off treatment won't suddenly bring you a new set of highlights. But it brightens the existing colour hugely. 'I always leave it till the last minute to book a colour appointment and my colourist is never free, so I spend a week or two desperately trying to cover up my roots,' admitted Pauline (47). 'This little miracle genuinely helped me through the bad hair days. It doesn't reinstate colour, but it has such a good clarifying effect on your hair, the roots don't seem to be so bad.'

the science bit: the magic ingredient is apparently vitamin C, which revitalises your hair's colour brightness and gloss. There are three parts to the treatment: you mix a powder into a lotion, apply it and leave it on for five minutes. Then you rinse and apply the conditioning treatment, leaving that on for five to ten minutes.

Kerastase Age Recharge

£14.95 for 150ml

There is a growing trend for 'anti-ageing' hair care products (it was only a matter of time), and while we are not convinced that these are ever going to take off in quite the same way as anti-ageing face creams, some of them – if judged on their own merit and this product included – are extremely effective. 'I've never used a mask before,' said Jane (67). 'I've never felt the need for one and I don't usually have the time. But I gave this a try and it really made me think again because it greatly improved the feel and texture of my hair. It felt thicker, my colour even looked brighter, and my hair was very silky and soft.' Our advice is to use this for its conditioning boost – not its 'anti-ageing' benefits: all hair can lose its lustre no matter how old you are.

the science bit: contains a reparative Vita-Ressource Complexe plus Euphorbia wax, shine-boosting soluble silicones and the anti-oxidant vitamin E. The mask should be worked into towel-dried hair a section at a time, left for five minutes then well rinsed out.

Know How Smoothing Moisture-Deep Treatment

£5.99 for 125ml

Aims either to smooth or volumise hair – a simple formula really, but we like that. It doesn't work as quickly as some conditioners, but it promises deeper conditioning – and we don't think you can expect results like these in a minute. It works on all hair types, so it will calm down mega curly hair or hair which is basically straight but has a lot of frizz – perhaps because it has been colour treated. 'Seemed to feel quite refreshing on my scalp,' said a smoother-haired Victoria (33). 'It smells of Moroccan mint tea. And it made my hair so soft afterwards it looked great with minimal styling.'

the science bit: contains aloe barbadensis leaf juice taken from the aloe plant which has moisturising properties, and micronised marine extracts which are said to maintain moisture in the hair shaft. Apply and leave on towel-dried hair for five minutes before rinsing out.

hair styling products

Where do we begin?! If you think it's daunting to be faced with row upon row of hair styling gels, mousses, creams and sprays in the chemist or supermarket, try rounding them up and finding out which ones work best for a book – it's a complete killer!

Of all the product categories we tested this was the one that filled us with the most dread: day after day styling products arrived in the post and had to be found homes. We had boxes full of defining and shining silicone-based serums, hairsprays (light, medium and extra hold), straightening and anti-frizz balms, thickening lotions and curl enhancers.

'if you have slicked your hair with gel and it starts to lose its shape don't add more product: wet your fingertips and run them through your hair to resculpt it'

Like many beauty products – especially anti-ageing creams and make-up – hair styling products are driven by trends that are decided by the market or inspired by the catwalks. Which is fine. Except not everyone wants their hair to look like it has been styled for a performance on *Pop Idol*, or has the time to turn the ends into flat spikes.

Some of us just want products that make our hair easier to straighten, bigger and with more lift – from the roots up – or even just less flyaway and fluffy after washing.

So we based our road-test criteria on more practical styling products for women like ourselves who mostly want to make their hair look *good* rather than making a fashion statement everyday. The fruits of our labours – and our testers' work – are all here.

what makes a good hair styling product?

1. Generally speaking, **the more lightweight the better**: if styling products are too heavy they will weigh your hair down and make it look dull.
2. **One which can be used sparingly**: less is definitely more in this case.
3. **One which is easy to use**: if it's too much of a pfaff you won't bother to use it – unless you are a teenager and have all the time in the world to play with your hair.

... hair styling products we rate:

Julia Charles Worthington Looks Amazing Invisible Control Blow-Dry Spray (£4.99 for 150ml) and Charles Worthington Results Stay In Shape Hair Super-spray (£3.99 for 200ml): 'I swap around with these when I'm blow-drying my own hair. They hold a style but they don't seem to make your hair look all stiff and formal. They also have a nice light scent.'

Kate Citre Shine Get Smooth Straightening Balm (£4.95 for 100ml): 'Despite writing about beauty for years I didn't get to grips with styling my own hair until recently. It's fine, thick and quite curly, so straightening it is a tall order for a styling gel. But this product – together with a lot of arm wrestling with a hairdryer and brush – works without making my hair greasy and lank the following day.'

the 8 best hair-styling products

the mission to find you the most effective and user-friendly hair styling products on the market.

the criteria our testers judged the styling products they tried on their ability to control hair and a style, add shape, texture, volume and definition without weighing hair down or making it look lank. They also tested hair styling products for their smell, and whether they were good value for money.

L'Oréal FX Architect Wax £3.99 for 75ml

This wax is best for short- to mid-length hair – and great if you happen to have a lot of layers that you want to chunk up, or to define a long wispy fringe. Catherine (40) has a cute short crop, and thought this wax gave her cut really good definition and texture. She commented: 'It's half-wax half-gel, so it feels lighter and less greasy than ordinary waxes. It absorbed well leaving my hair silky, not slimy, and well structured.' Because it isn't all wax it doesn't leave your hands feel tacky after applying it and you can keep adding more to your hair without it becoming overloaded. We think the best way to use it is to rub a little into your fingertips to warm it up like putty, then apply it to your hair.

Aveda Brilliant Humectant Pomade £15 for 75ml

This has to be one of the most pleasant smelling hair products around – in fact the entire Aveda range smells gorgeous (one of our testers said if she could she would just buy Aveda beauty products for this reason), giving the feeling of really fresh, clean hair – a major plus point for us and our testers. Look in most hairstylist's kitbags and you will see this little blue pot of pomade – for a reason. It seems to work on all hair types, giving styles precision and hair shine; and it keeps frizz to a minimum very well (listen up all those testers who asked us to find them a product that would do this and maintain the effects even when it rains). 'It's the only product that doesn't look like I've put a load of gunk in my hair, and it lets me style it exactly how I want it,' said Debbie (30).

Paul Mitchell Dry Wax

£8.95 for 50g

Another non-sticky or greasy wax which works on all hair lengths, but especially shorter styles (in fact it turned out to be quite a hit with some of our tester's other halves), and it helps to keep the shape or a particular style in place. Also works well on curls – giving them definition without taking the shine off hair; this can be a problem with curly hair and styling waxes. 'It's a bit of an all-rounder really,' said Claire (42). 'No heavy texture and just a little bit was all I needed to sort my wayward fringe out. I found it works very well on my eyebrows too!' Thanks for the tip.

Nicky Clarke Colour Therapy Move ME Mousse

£4.99 for 150ml

Our aim is to be honest, so we have to say that there were very few – if any – hair styling products that our testers really thought enhanced the colour of their highlighted or coloured hair. What they did find though was that some made their hair look brighter and shinier, so making the existing colour look better. And this mousse – which should be worked through the roots and ends of towel-dried hair and comes in four colours – was the best at giving these benefits. But both of our blonde testers said that the best thing about it is that it made their hair wonderfully soft and genuinely more manageable. One of them, Sal (24), has lots of highlights and describes her hair as 'straw-like'. 'I like it like that,' she said. 'But it's nice to have it feel soft sometimes too. This mousse did exactly that but it didn't make my hair go flat. I even told my hairdresser about it.'

Over The Top Self Raising Lotion Blow Dry Volumizer

£11.50 for 175ml

This lotion aims to add extra oomph to thin, lifeless hair without making it dry, limp or difficult to brush – something that tends to be a problem with some spray-in thickeners. The difference is that this is a heat-activated volumiser, so it needs to be applied to warm, towel-dried hair, and contains ingredients – including proteins – that add volume and moisture. Helena (28) has shoulder-length hair that is a little thin on the ground. She said, 'I've never heard of this make before, but the product had a nice smell, didn't feel sticky on my hair and seemed to make blow-drying easier. My hair looked great afterwards, not so flyaway and definitely had more weight to it.'

Citré Shine Get Smooth Straightening Balm

£4.95 for 100ml

We were amazed at how many of our testers thought that all they had to do with hair straightening balms, gels and creams was to put the product on – and not bother blow-drying or using straightening irons – and their hair would automatically straighten itself. If only life were that simple! Having said that, this balm seems to make the whole boring straightening process as easy as it can be because although you need a drier to get the best results you don't necessarily need straightening irons. 'My hair needs a lot of help to make it look smooth,' said wavy-haired Louise (32). 'And I don't like using irons on it all the time for fear of damaging it. This worked just as well – if not better – than the expensive one I'm used to, and which does need blow-drying with a brush and straightening irons. I'll definitely be buying it from now on.'

Umberto Giannini Glossing Mist

£2.95 for 75ml

It is so easy to make your hair look greasy when you use a serum or shine spray – it comes out so quickly – so the usual advice is to apply a small amount of the spray-on versions to your hands first and then to your hair. However, this mist seems to be so light that you can get away with spritzing it straight onto your hair. Joy (63) loves this spray – and especially the mini handbag version. She said, 'It's a nice fine mist and very light so it didn't add any unwanted weight to my hair. My hair is naturally very curly – I like to keep it straight – and quite dry too, but this managed to give it a healthy-looking sheen without my curls popping back.'

John Frieda Frizz Ease Serum

£5.95 for 50ml

The best-selling high performance hair serum for frizzy hair: so many women (and lots of our testers) use this product, its qualities cannot be ignored. Its formula allows it to repel moisture – thus making it so good at reducing frizziness (another good solution for those whose hair goes frizzy in the rain); it contains an ultra-violet (UV) sunscreen and there are different formulas for different types of hair – including original, medium frizz and Afro hair. 'I use it because it tames my hair,' wrote Georgiana (21). 'My hair is straight but I still use it to calm the static and de-fluff my split ends,' said Michelle (32), and Toni (31) simply wrote 'just brilliant' on her questionnaire. We think it is best applied when your hair is still wet because it distributes more evenly, and you only need a tiny amount – you can always add more after you have blow-dried your hair. (You need to apply quite a lot to push hair over the 'clean' boundary and into greasy.)

the 2 best setting sprays

L'Oréal Elnett Hairspray £3.69 for 200ml

Over 40 years old and there is still very little out there to match the performance of this hair spray. Used by all hairstylists, this was the world's first lacquer-free hair-spray (which basically means it fixes hair without giving it that 'set' look and can be easily brushed out) and it contains satin conditioners to give hair softness 'I just know I can trust it,' wrote Jane (67), 'I wouldn't bother trying anything else.' It now comes in different variants to cater for all hair types and conditions – from Supreme Hold to Extra Strength with Nutri-Ceramide for Dry or Damaged Hair.

Pure Hair Sandal Wood Finishing Spray £10.50 for 250ml

'I use lots of hairspray, so it's good to have a big can of the stuff, and I know I'll use all of this because it works very well. It's got a nice smell and I found that you can keep applying it without your hair going crispy,' said Emma (44). Some people hate the smell of hairspray and the way it collects in your throat – some of our testers admitted that they could not use Elnett for this reason. This is a great spray, but it also smells gorgeous (probably because of the essential oils it has in it – including moisturising clary – and lack of artificial fragrance); it also has a non-aerosol dispenser and a UV filter.

'frizzy, fluffy hair? Mix some hair gel with some serum and apply to your hair: the serum with stop the gel stiffening as it dries, stop hair frizzing and boost shine'

MAKE-UP

What do you think when you put on your make-up? (apart from worrying about being late for the school run or the office): that your 'look' seems to be morphing into your mother's? That you need a new mascara because the one you are using has dried up (not surprisingly as you have had it for a year)? Or that you still aren't convinced that your foundation is the right colour even though you have used up half the pot?

It usually comes down to time, but it must be said that make-up takes a back seat for many of us. Sure, we love a new mascara or lipgloss every now and then – but they are a pretty 'safe' buy anyway, because you can't really go too far wrong with them. What we are not good at though is getting the basics sorted – make-up like blusher and everyday lipstick, which underpin a look and which you should not even have to think about because they fit like a glove – and regularly reviewing the cosmetics we use.

Apart from finding the time, our biggest problem is choice. Being faced with such an alarming selection of cosmetics makes shopping for make-up very off-putting. And it doesn't help when you are chased up and down the counter by an assistant wielding the latest line-zapping 3D primer (which you probably don't need anyway).

So where do you start?

With the basics. You need to find your dream foundation – one that was made for *you* (be it a tinted moisturiser, compact base, fluid or mousse) – the most perfect blusher, a good brow pencil, mascara and lip colour. Once you have got the make-up you know you can rely on to make you look great (no matter how *un*great you *feel*) you can experiment confidently with other cosmetics. Just remember to review things every year or so.

In this section we will show you how to work out what cosmetics you need – and which ones perform best – so you can confidently go to a counter and buy them, with the least amount of fuss and without being sidetracked into buying stuff you don't need.

This is the honest make-up advice you have been waiting for.

What you will find out about in this chapter:

- Which cosmetic instantly shaves ten years off your face
- Why glittery lipgloss and pale iridescent lipstick deserve to go in the bin
- Why it is usually *your fault* if mascara sticks your lashes together
- Which nail varnish colour makes stubby fingers look longer and slimmer
- What kind of foundation makes *everyone's* skin look fantastic
- Why nothing dates a face faster than eyeshadow
- Why putting matt concealer on your face can be as bad as sticking a plaster on it

foundations

If you want to know how to get yourself the best foundation your money can buy you are reading the right book because we absolutely LOVE the stuff! We are both big foundation wearers and have very strong ideas about what makes a great base. There is, after all, no point wearing foundation unless it is great.

'how do you know when you have the right foundation? When you can't see it'

The only thing we agree to differ on is how much you need to spend on it. Julia doesn't think you need to splash out to get a good one because she – as well as, it seems, a lot of the women who tested products for us – has always found that the cheaper ones perform well. Kate, on the other hand, thinks you should spend money on foundation because the more expensive ones have always worked best for her.

What we can categorically say is that foundation does more for your skin than any other cosmetic: quite simply, if you haven't got good skin, the right foundation will make it good. It will also take years off your face – not put them on as a lot of people mistakenly believe. In fact if you think foundation will make your face look all powdery like your grandmother's you clearly haven't used it in a very long time!

Foundation formulas are so clever now (actually make that ingenious!): they care for your skin as well as making it look great, protect it from ultraviolet (UV) rays and moisturise it. Many contain active anti-ageing properties and some change colour with the light so your skin is always seen in the most flattering way.

So is it possible to get one that has the right benefits and finish – and comes in a colour that suits your skin? It *so* is! Just read on to find out how.

how to find the foundation that was made for you

This question was right up there with 'do anti-ageing creams really work?' on our survey response sheets. It was asked time and time again. So all those who asked will be interested to hear that there *is* a science to the search. Follow these steps and we *guarantee* you will end up with a base that looks as if it was made-to-measure:

1. Decide when you are going to wear the foundation – evenings only, or during the day when you are likely to need a more durable base.
2. Decide what kind of coverage you want – sheer or medium (few foundations give heavy coverage now – even the ones that are specially made to cover blemishes like port wine stains, vitiligo and scars).
3. Decide what kind of finish you want, bearing in mind that the most flattering finish for *all* skins (except very oily) is satin.
4. Decide how much you want to spend. This will probably dictate where you go to buy your foundation, but even if it's from a chemist you should try to test the base on your jaw-line – not your hand – before buying it. Most chemists don't have proper testing facilities which is very frustrating, and the only way around this is to carry a portable mirror with you.
5. Bring home a sample to try in natural light. Most beauty counters have sachets hidden away expressly for this purpose: all you have to do is ask.

five good reasons to wear foundation

If you have never worn it – and don't much fancy the idea of covering your face with foundation – consider these bonuses:

1. It makes your skin look flawless, smooth and even-textured – skin pigment irregularities and minor blemishes like broken veins will be less noticeable.
2. It helps make-up go on, last longer and look better – colours look smooth, not choppy.
3. It protects your skin from ultraviolet (UV) light – useful if your moisturiser doesn't contain a sun protection factor (SPF).
4. It moisturises your skin – and can even help to fight the signs of time, as some foundations contain active anti-ageing ingredients.
5. It can make your skin tighter, younger and plumper.

foundations with a specific purpose

Some faces need 'heavier' coverage to tone-down or soften (we hate the word hide when it comes to cosmetics) blemishes like port wine stains and scars, and high colour. Not long ago the only choices for this were thick, cakey bases which went on your face like a mask and looked totally unnatural. But they have been greatly improved – mainly by adding more colour pigment and silicones to the formulas (which means that even when used sparingly they cover very effectively) and enhancing their efficacy so they are easier and more pleasant to use. Find out which ones performed best in our road-test results (see pages 131–135).

how to choose the perfect finish

matt & ultra-matt – shine-free and long-lasting, foundations with this kind of finish suit people with an oily skin type best.
satin & demi-matt – halfway between matt and shine, foundations with this finish are the most flattering for all skins, especially mature.

can't decide which base to go for?

Take our advice: the most flattering foundation for *all skins* is a sheer, light-reflective one with a demi-matt or satin finish, it makes all skins – young and old – look fantastic. If you can get this in the right colour for your skin you can't go wrong.

never

- buy foundation without trying it: even if you don't want to ask for advice at a beauty counter (several of our testers said they won't do this because they know the advice is biased), it is worth asking for a sample of foundation
- wear a foundation that doesn't exactly match your skin colour
- wear pink, rose or peach coloured foundation because you have got pale skin
- wear oil-based foundation if you have got oily skin and oil-free or matt foundation if you haven't got oily skin
- apply too much – no matter how sheer the formula is, if you layer it on too thickly it will look like a mask
- apply foundation to warm skin – it will just melt and disappear

always

- apply foundation with your fingers or a brush, so much of it gets wasted inside sponges
- try foundation before you buy it
- apply foundation where you need it – most of us don't need it all over our faces
- take the application below your jaw and blend it into your neck
- blend it well around your hairline

what light-reflective foundation can do for you

Many people can't see the point of sheer foundations, saying they don't 'do anything' and can't be seen. But if they are light-reflective they do *a lot*, believe us, but subtly: make-up should emphasise the good and play down the not-so-good, and mirrored particles enhance this principle in two ways:

1. **it makes skin look better** because instead of being absorbed, reflective pigments bounce light off skin so flaws go into 'soft focus' and the complexion gets a more translucent luminosity than the flat 'warmth' created by regular bases.
2. **it enhances your features** because it magnifies and brightens.

five key foundation pointers

1. **think pigment:** pale skin often suits yellow-based foundations more than pink – a find made by MAC founder Frank Toscani. Dark skins need pigment-rich talc-free bases which don't make skin look ashen and can be used sparingly.
2. **think thin:** sheer bases do more for most skins than thick because they subtly even-out skin tone and imperfections rather than just covering everything up like a mask. Even better if they are light-reflective. All skins look better with less foundation – especially young and mature; and you can't substitute a crepy, wrinkled complexion with 'second skin' from a bottle, it looks fake.
3. **think healthy:** the aim is vibrant skin. A satin finish makes skin look fit and healthy (we are not talking about 'sweaty' here – the shiny directional look you sometimes see in magazines which doesn't work in real life), and light-play enhances the effect. Matt finish foundation tries to make a comeback every so often, but it will never be flattering for anyone over the age of 16. Matt bases make all skins except perhaps oily look flat, dry and old.
4. **think timing:** apply foundation at the right moment – soon after moisturising, when skin is supple and will accept it best. Put your foundation on by a window; natural light is unforgiving but truthful and reliable.
5. **think 'second skin':** unless you have got very oily skin use your fingers to apply fluid foundations so you can really blend it in well, especially around your nose, hair and jaw line; and only put it where it's needed – usually T-zone, sometimes cheeks, *rarely all over*. Use a brush to apply foundation to oily skin as fingers can deposit yet more grease on the surface.

shopping for foundation

Before you head for the shops or flash your cash:

1. **Sample the foundation.** If you can, take a sample home to try it on your face and away from shop lighting which can distort colour. If you can't, your only option is to try it on in the shop – on your jaw-line, *not* the back of your hand.
2. **Do some research** (i.e. read this chapter thoroughly!) into the kind of foundation finishes that will flatter your skin best.
3. **Decide how much you want to spend**: our testers found that foundations from across the board – cheap through to mid-range and premium – performed well, although a couple of testers, including Caroline (42) and Michelle (38), said that after testing foundations for us they realised it is worth spending a bit more if you want to get superlative results.

... foundations we rate:

Julia i.d BareMinerals Foundation (£24.50 for 9gm): 'This is a powder foundation with a matt-like finish which you put on with a brush in a few seconds. It's made of minerals, (so yes – you could sleep in it), it comes in 8 shades which you can blend to get the perfect tone, it's just the best, longest-lasting foundation I've found, and by far the easiest to apply.'

Kate Christian Dior Teint Dior Lift (£23 for 30ml): 'Dream texture, the best shades and a perfect satin finish. This foundation transforms your skin and the results have to be seen to be believed. I can't see myself ever using any other foundation.'

the 15 best foundations

the mission to find you the most effective and user-friendly foundations on the market.

the criteria our testers reviewed the foundations they tried on their ability to enhance their skin, cover minor blemishes and tonal irregularities. They also judged them on their application – how easy they are to put on, how well and long they lasted, how comfortable they are to wear, how realistic their colours are, what they smell like and whether they are good value for money.

Prescriptives Traceless Skin Response Tint Levels 1–6

£22 for 30ml

'So good on my very sensitive skin that I've now gone and bought the concealer and powder to match,' said Anne (42), one of the women who has tried this foundation and rated it highly. Heloise (31) wrote, 'They call it a skin tint and it's quite runny, but it still gives you the same effects as foundation. It's just very light. I think it's one of the best foundations I've tried. Fantastic.' The foundation has a high density of colour pigment in it so it gives skin good coverage without being like a mask. It is perfect for people who like a non-make-up look but still want to cover up blemishes.

the science bit: uses properties called Light Right Prisms – hi-tech light-reflectors which manipulate the impact of light on your skin, so it looks perfectly uniform.

Clinique Superfit

£17 for 30ml

Voted high by our testers for its all-round versatility, this is an 'anytime, anywhere kind of foundation' according to Helen (39) and suits all skin types. It has a good light consistency which feels substantial enough to give coverage where it is needed most. The formula is oil-free – so ideal for summer or if you have very oily skin – and it lasts well. Helen said she calls it her 'lazy make-up foundation' because she doesn't have to put too much effort into applying it to get good results. Lisa (37) commented that 'it stays put for most of the day, it's reliable'.

the science bit: the key properties in this base are microdernier nylon fibres which absorb excess oil, and pigments which have been treated so that colour stays true even when foundation comes into contact with oil and perspiration.

Clarins Multi-Matte Foundation

£17 for 30ml

Best for oily complexions – or if you have a particularly oily T-zone – this mattifying foundation keeps shine to a minimum. Amanda (40) said, 'Its most outstanding bonus is its resilience – it lasts very, very well and it feels comfortable to wear,' and Sue (42), added 'I found it had really good staying power – it stayed matt all day and didn't make my skin feel caked or clogged which it often does with foundation.'

the science bit: pigment is the key to this base; the key one – concelight – is coated in silicones which help it glide onto skin and absorb any oil or perspiration, keeping skin matt and the colour and coverage true.

Clarins Hydra-Balance Tinted Moisturiser

£19 for 50ml

A favourite of both of ours. In the days when neither of us had much clue about foundation or how to apply it, we both used this foundation, and still do in its newer form: this is an idiot-proof workhorse – it works really well every time you put it on and its creamy consistency gives just the right amount of coverage. 'I've used it for years,' said Michelle (32), 'to me it's the perfect texture; the shade I use – Blonde – seems to look right all year round. I love the fresh, clean smell and I'm just really happy with it.'

the science bit: contains potent hydrators and corrective pigments which even out your skin tone and make it look uniform.

Dermablend Cover Crème

£13.95 for 10.7gm

There is a very limited choice of foundations that give the kind of opaque coverage that is needed to conceal blemishes like port wine stains, birthmarks and scars. This was the one our testers who said they needed heavier coverage used and agreed was the most effective. 'Although it gives the heavy coverage you need it doesn't look or feel like a mask, which is what people expect,' said Emma (39). 'My problem is hyper-pigmentation, which I got when I was pregnant with my second baby, and has never completely gone. I use this like a concealer – just dotting it on where I need it (mostly my cheeks and my hairline) – and it works very well. Please tell people to try it in your book!'

the science bit: the key is the pigment – it is up to ten times richer than most commercial foundations and is developed to blend so easily it gives uniform results even if you only use it on certain areas of your face.

Maybelline Fresh Matte All-Day Foundation

£4.99 for 30ml

'It stayed matt all day and I have an oily T-zone,' said Angela (44). 'It's good, I'd buy it again.' Tina (56) said, 'I think the most amazing thing about this one is that it doesn't let your skin get shiny but it doesn't make it feel dry and tight too – like so many of them do. It's lovely to have skin that feels fresh and supple and looks brighter.'

the science bit: the key ingredient in this base is a lilac pigment which is what gives the foundation a special skin-brightening quality.

Bobbi Brown Foundation Stick

£26 for 9gm

On the whole, foundation sticks did not go down that well with our testers; they found them too drying or greasy and not easy enough to blend onto skin. This one seemed to fare very well though – despite the fact that a couple of people said it felt a bit greasy. 'It feels almost greasy when you apply it, but this makes it easier to blend and it doesn't look shiny or feel sticky when it's all on and smoothed into your skin,' said Sophie (31). Zoe (27) thought the colour she tried (the second palest shade in the range) was very good too: 'It just melted into my skin – I've never had that luck with foundation before – and I looked less tired. You can use it as concealer too, did you know?!'

the science bit: beeswax provides the 'slip' – so when the foundation goes on it glides easily over your skin, and a property called silica controls oil and shine.

No7 Ultimate Mousse Foundation

£11.50 for 30ml

Absolutely the best mousse foundation on the market – and a great price for a product that is not easy to manufacture. The colour pigments, UV-protective sunscreens and vitamin E all somehow manage to come out of the nozzle in foam form. 'I love this base,' said Katie (21). 'It's as light as air, and because it's a mousse it doesn't feel scary to apply – you know you won't make a mistake with it. The colours are good; I've used – name tbc [missing info] – on my skin for years, and the coverage is very sheer but effective.'

the science bit: a 'colour and care' foundation which evens up skin for its day job and treats your skin at the same time.

Chantecaille Real Skin SPF30

£39 for 11gm

A cult foundation (and a favourite with many beauty writers) with a lightweight gel-like consistency. The effects are extremely sheer, and we thought our testers would reject it for this reason, but it proved to be a complete hit. 'It's quite unique,' said Janey (47), 'well, I've never used anything like it before. You hardly need to look when you put it on because it's so easy to apply – you don't even feel like you are putting anything on your face – and it gives you a fresh, dewy effect. It seemed to me that the less of it you use the better the effects are.'

the science bit: a blend of micro-particle powders and oils, the formula excludes lanolin and mineral oil which some people claim to be sensitive to.

Almay Nearly Naked Touch Powder Compact Make Up

£8.99 for 15ml

We were amazed how many people liked the 'barely there' foundations we sent them – bases which are so lightweight and sheer you think they won't do anything but give surprisingly good coverage and uniformity to skin. Lily (51) flipped over this one: 'This is fantastic. Timesaving and effective,' she said, 'it gives your skin a light covering and it's the most effective foundation I've used since my old Dior one.'

the science bit: oil-free and, as with all Almay cosmetics, hypo-allergenic and fragrance-free.

Nivea Tinted Moisturising Crème

£6.65 for 50ml

A very simple tinted moisturiser which comes in just two shades – Natural, for fair skins and Bronze, for tanned or darker skins. Alice (40) and Philly (32) loved it. Alice said, 'It brightens your skin up, great in winter, doesn't "sit" on top of it looking unreal and blends in really easily.' Philly added, 'You don't have to worry about it when you've got it on because it doesn't feel heavy, you know it hasn't gone patchy and it's a good colour match. I used Natural.' Both think it is a great budget buy.

the science bit: clever use of colour and light-reflective pigments manipulate light to even out the skin's texture and tone.

Iman Second To None Cream to Powder Foundation

£21.90 for 0.3oz

This foundation comes in two formulas – the other one is oil-free, so ideal for oily or darker skin tones (which tend to be greasier than pale). This turned out to be a hit mainly because it is quick and simple to use. We feel it is at its best when you use it to cover just your T-zone or other areas, because it blends so brilliantly. 'Most cream-to-power foundations I've used before have needed powder on top to be honest,' said Caroline (42). 'This one didn't – and I'm fussy! It's got a light texture to it but actually gives quite opaque coverage, which is what I need.'

the science bit: contains pigments that match skin's undertones, one of the keys to getting colour right for darker skins. Available in 16 shades from fair to dark.

Max Factor Lasting Performance

£9.50 for 35ml

Fifteen thousand of these foundations are apparently sold every week in the UK – and we can see why: this is another face base our testers loved. 'Perfect coverage. It's just as good – if not better – than other expensive foundations I've tried,' commented Dierdre (38). It is lightweight, but still gives good coverage and manages to stay put and not end up in unwanted places (your collar, mobile phone, etc). 'I've been using this for a number of years now because I haven't found anything that compares in this price range. It's better than either of the other two you sent me,' said Lisa (39).

the science bit: its star benefit is a 'touch resistant system' which means it won't end up anywhere other than your face. So no migrating or smudging.

La Prairie Skin Caviar Foundation SPF15

£95 for 0.55gm

Alice (34) described this foundation as being like 'liquid velvet' – which is spot on. We both love it – it is one of the best liquid foundations we have tried, and the packaging alone is a work of art (although we were not testing foundations on their packaging). 'It gives your skin the most unbelievably gorgeous finish,' said Hilary (44), another convert. 'It is a luxury, but definitely worth it.' Kate thinks using this foundation is a bit like having a couture dress (except that she has never had one): once you have had one you can't go back to the high street. Ahh, bless!

the science bit: the formula includes caviar (yes, real caviar) which has nourishing and firming qualities, silica and a property called nylon 12, which scatters light helpfully and diminish the appearance of fine lines.

MAC Studio Tech Foundation

£22 for 10gm

A brilliant cream-to-powder base from a make-up range that has been incredibly well thought up – by a make-up artist, Frank Toscani. The big point of difference for MAC foundations is a yellow pigment that makes them incredibly well suited to fair and oriental skin tones. This foundation has a good creamy texture, so it blends well and gives light to medium coverage and a demi-matt (satin) finish. Sara (22) said, 'I'd never dream of spending this much on a foundation in my normal life. But as I've worked my way through the pot I've decided I would be prepared to save up and buy this one. I suffer with spots and this is the first foundation I've used which has given me real confidence because I know I don't have to keep retouching it.'

the science bit: apart from its unique colour matching abilities, this base offers light-reflective qualities which can make skin look younger and fresher.

concealers

You either love concealer or would rather run up a mountain than wear it. If you do use it, we think it pays to be a snob about it because, like foundation, there is no point owning, let alone wearing, a concealer that doesn't perform miracles. Unless you want to exaggerate the problem. Which is exactly what most of us end up doing because we don't use concealers that are the right colour, consistency or finish, and just put it on 'blemishes' – anything from dark under-eye circles to spots – without thinking that it might not have been developed for this particular problem.

'spot cover is not the same as concealer for dark undereye circles'

One concealer can't magic away everything because different blemishes need a different coverage: covering a spot, for instance, is quite different to covering dark shadows. Besides, if you aim to conceal something completely it invariably looks worse; whereas 'softening' or 'diffusing' a blemish tends to be more successful.

There is no doubt that concealer is a useful little staple to have in your bathroom cabinet – as long as it's the right one. Here's how to find it.

which concealer do you need?

The kind of concealer you buy depends on the imperfection you want to play down – the concealer you keep for zapping spots is not likely to work on your dark under-eye shadows (which is why Caroline, in answer to your question, the concealer you are using is falling into the lines under your eyes!). So it is important to get the right concealer for the right job:

- **dark shadows** under and at the inside corners of eyes need softening with light cream concealers such as those sold in tubes, mini pots or as brush-tip pens. The best are light-reflective (they ping light away from dark zones and brighten the area up) and have a demi-matt finish. It's important too that any concealer you use around your eye is rich in colour pigment, so you can use the smallest amount to the greatest effect. Always apply under-eye concealer with a brush.
- **spots** need cream-to-powder concealers like the stick ones that come in swivel-up tubes like lipsticks, compacts or wand applicators, with a high pigment density. If the skin around the spots is dry and flaky you may be better off with a cream demi-matt finish concealer.
- **lines** – fine and deep (like mouth-to-nose naso-labials which can look deeper and red when you are tired) – can be 'softened' with demi-matt cream concealers such as those that come in tubes or brush-tip pens which make them easier to apply accurately. They should have a demi-matt finish and contain light-reflective particles to diffuse the line and make it look less obvious by illusion.
- **scars** and blemishes like birthmarks and port wine stains need specific concealers which are extremely high in pigment – and provide thicker coverage – to disguise them. In recent years these concealers have improved no end and there are two good ranges available in the UK: Keromask, which came out best in our concealer road tests, and Dermablend, which fared well in foundations.
- **tattoos** can be covered, but it is worth remembering from the outset that you may not manage to conceal them 100 percent.

never

- use concealer that dries to a matt powder on any part of your face – under your eyes, over spots or lines, anywhere – it's as bad as wearing a plaster.
- wear yellow, mauve, apricot or green 'colour correctors' and concealers – these were made for aliens not humans, and no one other than make-up artists working with studio or theatre lighting can put them on properly.
- apply concealer too quickly over eye cream or moisturiser – it will migrate and streak or slip into deeper lines and highlight them for the world to see.
- use a concealer that is darker than your skin – even if you are desperate; it should be one shade lighter than your skin.

beauty scoop highly commends:

- Dermablend Leg & Body Cover (£19.95 for 64gm) – highly pigmented, long wearing and waterproof (so it serves you on the beach too), it covers tattoos, birthmarks, port wine stains, scars, big moles and burns.

shopping for concealers

Before you head for the shops or flash your cash:

1. Decide what you want the concealer for – spots, under-eye bags, lines or more obvious scars and blemishes.
2. Decide what form of concealer will be most practical for you to use – cream, solid cream in a compact, brush-on or twist-up like a lipstick.
3. Decide how much you want to spend: a couple of concealers from the more competitive brands got the thumbs up from our testers.

... concealers we rate:

Julia i.d Bare Escentuals Eye Colour (£12): 'I use this in a shade called Bisque as concealer because I think it does the job brilliantly – especially on my dark circles. I've also been trying the concealer inside the lid of La Prairie Skin Caviar Beauté a Porter Concealer/Foundation SPF15 (£65 for 2.5ml) which is prohibitively expensive, but so, so good. It blends so beautifully – like silk!

Kate 'I don't use concealer. I rely totally on foundation, especially if my skin is looking ropey.'

the 5 best concealers

the mission to find you the most effective and user-friendly concealers on the market.

the criteria our testers judged the concealers they tried on their ability to cover minor facial imperfections like dark circles, broken veins and red scars. They also reviewed the colour ranges, ease of application and resilience.

Laura Mercier Secret Camouflage

£24 for 7.7gm

The beauty editor's secret weapon: this concealer, developed by leading make-up artist Laura Mercier, was one of the first that used the high pigment concept – which means a little goes a long way, and that blemishes can be covered very easily and sparingly. It comes in a palette with two shades – light and dark – that can be mixed together to make the perfect one for your skin. Fi (38) said 'I wasn't sure about it at first – I thought it looked a bit cakey and would show. I'm not a big concealer fan anyway. But the thing about it is that you only need the tiniest amount – it's amazing, it goes such a long way and covers up everything so well. I like the way you can mix the shades too because most concealers only come in colours the manufacturer decides to make and you don't have enough of a choice.'

the colours: six palettes each with two tones available.

Yves Saint Laurent Touche Eclat

£21 for 2.5ml

Probably the most famous concealer in the world – and undoubtedly the best-selling one – there can't be many people who haven't tried this magic light-reflective brush. It is a pump-action applicator that squeezes concealer out onto its brush so you can literally paint over dark under-eye circles and redness. So many of our testers said they used this product it almost deserved a category of its own. Annie (26) summed up everyone's remarks best when she said, 'I can't imagine not having it in my bag.' Enough said.

the colours: just the one suit-all flesh shade.

Body Shop Lightening Touch

£8 for 7ml

Some people call this the poor man's Touche Eclat, but Clare (40) said, 'It's just as good if not better and a fraction of the cost.' Julia is a big fan of this concealer too – she has used it for years and agrees with Clare's thoughts. There are no clever packaging or application gimmicks, Lightening Touch is dispensed on a plain sponge-tipped applicator so it can be blended with a (clean) fingertip, and the results are extremely good. Its light-reflective properties conceal and lift, so it works well on areas where there is darkness or redness – like around your nostrils and on deep lines.

the colours: two shades – 01 and 02.

Rimmel Hide The Blemish

£2.99 for 4.5gm

This one got the thumbs up for its spot-concealing benefits: 'It works so well on angry red spots,' said Paula (20), 'normally I don't bother to try and cover them up because it never really works – in fact it often makes the problem look worse. But this was more successful at it than any other concealer I've used.' It has a heavier consistency than many concealers, so it is best for covering spots and scars, not dark circles or large areas where it needs a lot of blending. Caroline (31) said, 'I've used it for years and have no plans to stop. It works really well.'

the colours: four colours from pale to dark.

Keromask Camouflage Cream £9.95 for 15ml

Far and away the best concealer for problems such as hyperpigmentation, vitiligo or port wine stains. Keromask is ten times more concentrated than regular concealers – so its pigment density is much higher and it covers problems like these very well without needing to be retouched for at least six hours. It can also work well on rosacea as long as the skin is not dry and red. 'I've got scars that will be with me forever unfortunately,' Marina (52) told us. 'I'm very conscious of them. This is my saviour. I discovered it a couple of years ago and it changed my life.' Sue (40) uses it to cover some acne scarring:'The reason it does this better than regular concealer is that it's so highly pigmented. You just "push" the pigment into your skin like a primer and blend it. It smoothes out acne scars very very well.'

the colours: four pre-mixer shades – ultra light, light, medium and dark, and five 'primaries' to mix them with.

blushers

Blusher had been sidelined for years until it came back into fashion recently. Make-up articles never really mentioned it because there didn't seem to be much to say other than to choose a pink one if you had fair skin and terracotta if you had dark.

Another reason why blusher has been ignored for so long is its association with two past (it) looks: old-fashioned slap – grandma's powdery face with lopsided splodges of pink on each cheek; and 1980s overkill (think *Dallas* and *Dynasty*) – the way Boy George and Steve Strange used fuschia blusher in this era was enough to put us all off it for life.

But blusher plays a very different role today.

We have finally woken up to the fact that it is one of the most important cosmetics you can own because it does much more than just add colour to your face: blusher literally transforms you face – it adds life to it and knocks years off it.

> 'don't match blusher to your lipstick – it's as naff as matching lips and nails'

Since its renaissance, blusher is now available in an infinite choice of refined colours from flesh pink to freckle, and blusher formulas are mostly very good: whether powder or cream, and applied by fingers or brush, the pigments tend to glide over your skin and are much easier to blend, which makes for a much more realistic flush.

We are not saying it's impossible to buy a bad blusher these days or that it is foolproof. But if you get it right, blusher is the easiest cosmetic to wear and – along with foundation – probably the most valuable in terms of what it can do for you.

cream or powder blusher?

We think this comes down to personal preference (Kate prefers creams, Julia powders). But if you have dry skin, cream or gel blushers may well work better for you than powder ones, and vice versa for oily skin. Powder blushers can make your face look more 'made-up' (and possibly older) than creams, so this is something to think about. If you do a job where appearances matter – but you don't have to look like a fashion plate everyday – powder blusher may be best. If you have dry, mature skin and like more casual make-up, you might find a cream blusher suits you better.

how to get the right colour blusher

This is key – the colour of blusher you wear can be the decider between a youthful, healthy face and a dated, tired one. This is likely to be the only occasion (other than choosing eye-shadow) you will hear us suggest you ignore fashion: blusher colours go in and out of fashion with every new catwalk show – sometimes mauve (and lots of it) is all the rage, and sometimes a hint of pink is hip. Let it go. The important thing is to wear a blusher that suits you, regardless of the trends.

Our tips on choosing the right colour are:

- avoid blushers which are very pale pink – they make you look like a ghost
- be wary of peach – it makes most skins look sallow
- give mauve a wide berth – it makes olive and pale skin look ashen
- try earthy shades like deep beige and golden brown if you have dark skin
- try blue-based pinks and flesh tones if you have pale skin – a hint of shimmer in these will 'lift' your face
- if in doubt use your naturally heightened skin colour as your guide – blusher should be the colour you go when you are naturally flushed

'the darker your skintone the more pigment-rich your blusher needs to be'

how to apply blusher

1. Blusher should go on after you have applied foundation – but before powder and any eye or lip colours – because it sets the 'canvas' for colour. You should put it straight onto foundation, not over powder. (Few people need to powder their whole faces anyway and even less their cheeks).
2. Apply blusher to the *top centre* of your cheekbones. If you are putting powder blusher on with a brush, start with a dusting (it's easier to add more than remove it) and build up the colour if you need to. Dust in tiny circles, making sure the colour is on the upper cheekbones – don't be tempted to bring it down further and make a bigger colour impact or to sweep it out to your hairline. Apply cream or gel blusher with a finger and blend it in circular movements, graduating more to the outer corner of your eye than below cheekbones.

types of blusher

- **powder blusher** works for all skin types; it comes pressed – sometimes with light-reflective pigments in it and even sparkling gold particles – and should be applied with a big soft brush. The only drawback to powder blusher is that it can 'sit' on your skin rather unnaturally, especially if it's applied to bare skin.
- **liquid, gel, cream, stick and cream-to-powder blushers** give more of a natural 'glow-from-within' look by virtue of the fact that they are not powder-based and tend to be absorbed a little by your skin. You use your fingers to apply them and we think they are easier to blend in than powder blushers (although the gels and liquids are harder), and suit skins which are not too oily or dry best.

never

- wear any other colour blusher than the one that looks like your natural flush – this is your guideline to choosing the right shade
- apply blusher in stripes from your cheekbones to your hairline
- use blusher to 'contour' your face or 'give yourself' cheekbones
- wear blusher on any part of your face other than your cheekbones

shopping for blusher

Before you head for the shops or flash your cash:

1. Decide whether you want a cream or powder blusher.
2. Work out which colour blusher is likely to suit you – pinkier tones or more earthy browns and beiges: the aim is to get the same colour as you would go when blushing naturally.
3. Decide how much you want to spend: it turned out that our testers liked blushers in the mid-range to premium brackets best.

... blushers we rate:

Julia Lancôme Blush Focus (£13): 'On minimal make-up days, all I need is a dot of this cream blusher for impact, and the range of colours is fabulous for all year round.'

Kate Clinique Natural Blush Blushwear (£12.50): 'My skin is so pale if I don't wear blusher I look like I'm about to pass out, so I always wear it even if I'm not wearing any other make-up. This is an easy-to-blend cream, the colour is the most natural I've found, and it seems to go on and on forever.'

the 6 best blushers

the mission to find you the most effective blushers and user-friendly blushers on the market.

the criteria our testers judged the blushers they tried on their colours – how realistic and true they are, their finish, ease of application and blendability, their staying-power and value for money.

Benefit Benetint £21.50

A break-away blusher – this was one of the first waterproof liquid tints, and it is clearly still the best. Being such a thin fluid, its main benefit is that it looks so natural because you can't see a layer of colour on the skin as you might with other cream blushers. It is the same colour as blood, so it can be a bit off-putting to use, but once dotted onto the apples of your cheeks and blended in it gives a very realistic flush. It works especially well on dark and olive skins. Lucy (27) said: 'I'm not a big make-up wearer – and I wouldn't dream of wearing blusher normally, which is why I love this. You have to get the hang of putting it on, but it's so fine it looks completely natural. You can stain your lips with it too.'

the colours: available in four shades – three pinky ones and one peach.

Shu Uemura Blusher £14

Popular with professional make-up artists, this blusher comes in an incredible selection of shades and because it has such strong pigment and fine texture it applies like a dream and goes a long way even when used very sparingly. 'I was recommended a shade I never would have thought would suit me when I went to Shu Uemura,' said Charlotte (39), 'it's a sort of orangey-brown and I'm fair skinned. But I couldn't believe how well it worked and how flattering. I'd buy it again, but not for ages because it seems to go on and on. Great buy.'

the colours: currently 30 non-shimmery shades.

Bobbi Brown Cream Blush Stick £18

'The thing I like most about this blusher is that you can't overdo the colour,' wrote Rachel (36). 'It's got a lovely creamy texture, so blending it in is effortless, and you can't overload the layers. I need a foolproof blusher because I've gone out so often and caught a glimpse of myself looking bright pink. I get a bit carried away.' This blusher can be applied directly to your cheeks or to fingertips first and then blended in to create a healthy-looking flush.

the colours: eight of them – including Desert Rose (great for pale skins), Sienna (the one for dark skins) and Coral (oriental skins).

Marks & Spencer Autograph Cheek Colourwash £10

Make-up artist Sharon Dowsett was the brains behind this make-up range for M&S, and her professional touch is evident in this blusher. A cream to powder in a little pot, it feels quite powdery to touch, but is very light and blends beautifully, leaving a matt finish. Joanna (25) said, 'It's very good value because you don't need much – it's obviously very highly pigmented, so it would last you a long time.' She went on to say she thought it made her look like 'a real English Rose'.

the colours: ten shades including one called Natural.

Blisslabs Glows £15

This blusher has a light, creamy texture, and as you apply it it turns to powder – which seems to make it easier to blend, so it is ideal for blusher novices. 'It's best described as creamy with a powdery edge to it,' said Louise (32), 'and it comes in some really good, flattering shades.' Hilary (44) said, 'It didn't sit on my skin and make me look like a doll or puppet which a lot of blusher seems to do. I've been put off blusher but this could persuade me back onto it.'

the colours: ten fab natural shades – Delicate is perhaps the best all-rounder.

Ruby & Millie Face Gloss £12

This is a blusher on push-up stick which is multi-purpose – you can also use on your lips and eyes to 'lift' all your features in a very natural way. 'I felt like I should be putting it in my hair or something – not on my cheeks – it's like one of those highlighting pens,' said Lorna (28). 'It looks a bit greasy at first, but it works brilliantly, giving just enough colour and a hint of healthy sheen.'

the colours: four shades – two dark ones called Wine (red based) and Tan (brown) plus Flush (pinky) and Fire (coral).

eye make-up

Eye shadow used to be much more integral to make-up than it is today. Most of us don't even bother with it in the day now; we get by on mascara and a little eye pencil definition, keeping eyeshadow for evenings or special occasion make-up. We think part of the reason for this is the perception that eyeshadow is high maintenance: you think it can't just be put on like blusher and forgotten about.

'don't wear more than two eyeshadows: the rainbow effect went out with the ark (except in the beauty halls of some department stores)'

But eyeshadow formulas have really improved over the past decade or so. Whether pressed powder, cream-to-powder or cream they are much more durable – cosmetic scientists have improved their 'cling factor' greatly; they go on more easily and come in softer, more realistic shades, so if they do smudge it's less noticeable. Besides, eyeshadow isn't the only make-up for your eyes. A single stroke of eye khol or pencil can be as effective at defining your eyes.

You don't need to be wearing the latest acid yellow eyeshadow to have a good, up-to-date look. What you need is eye make-up that suits your life style. Which is where we come in. We have spent months looking for eye make-up which we think is worthy of your hard-earned cash: eyeshadows that don't crease, khol which goes on evenly no matter how shaky your hands and soft pencils which won't drag your skin but are tough enough not to come off on your brow bones.

Read on to get the knowledge.

what eyeshadow can do for you

- Make your eye colour stronger
- Clarify and brighten the whites of your eyes
- Make your eyes look bigger, less droopy, close, wide or deep set
- Enhance the shape of your eyes
- Influence the overall appearance of your face

how to apply eyeshadow

If lack of skill is the only thing stopping you from wearing eyeshadow try this:

1. Make sure there is no oil – either natural sebum or moisturiser – on your lids.
2. Using a neutral tone – beige, soft brown, grey or khaki – apply a stroke of shadow to your lids from the outside corner in. Apply powder shadow with a long-handled brush (the best place for those mini applicators that come with eyeshadows is in the bin because you can never grip them properly), and cream or cream-to-powder shadow with a fingertip.
3. Blend away hard edges: your aim is for 'fuzzy definition'.

This is eyeshadow at its most basic. You can also use it to:

- **enlarge small eyes** by applying a medium shadow halfway across the lid from the outer corner to the inner, doing the same with eyeliner (on upper lids only) and lining the inside of your lower lids with a white eye pencil.
- **open out deep set eyes** by doing the same but using a darker shadow on the outer corners and drawing a (fuzzy) line across the whole of the upper lids as close to the lash-line as possible.
- **re-balance close-set eyes** by applying a light shadow on the inside corner of your lids and blending it with a dark shadow on the outside corners.
- **re-balance wide-set eyes** by doing the same as above but the other way around.

eye make-up rules for every woman

- **Less is more**: too much eyeshadow piles years on your face no matter how old.
- **Regularly update it**: not just when you get married, divorced or have a milestone birthday – and experiment with different shades and brands.
- **Watch the finish**: powder eyeshadows with a matt finish are less likely to highlight lines around your eyes but they can have quite a flat, chalky effect, while a hint of iridescence in a cream, cream-to-powder or powder shadow can 'lift' and brighten eyes – and soften fine lines near them.
- **Think natural**: eyeshadow tones that need lots of blending are wrong for you – the right ones will just seem to 'melt' into your skin.

high speed eye definition

eye pencils come in all shapes and sizes now – stubby little crayons, long elegant pencils (does anyone ever get to the end of these we wonder?) and twist-up pencils with waxy coloured nibs. They are great for high-speed eye definition.

Our tip: when it comes to choosing eye pencils get the softest you can find – it should glide over your skin almost without you feeling it (and definitely without dragging it); so always try it on your wrist before you buy it.

liquid eye khol can be easier on your eyes, but trickier to use – wobbly lines spoil the impact! The definition can also be quite hard – something few but the youngest faces can take well – and can't be softened up like eye pencil with a Q-tip.

Our tip: try to keep the line as smooth and close to your upper lash-line as possible. Try a soft shade like grey or brown first as black can be quite unforgiving, and use the felt-tip pen variety rather than a brush and liquid.

eyebrow pencils seem to be multiplying by the dozen ever since eyebrows came back into focus. Use them to fill in gaps between your brow hairs and extend the tail-end of your brows.

Our tip: get a brow pencil in a shade lighter than your hair colour (so get a beige one if you are a blonde or brunette and a brown one if you have black hair), and build up the effect slowly; it only takes a few strokes to overdo it and this kind of boob is a nightmare to reverse. If you have lost a lot of brow hairs and find you are drawing in most of your eyebrows you are better off with brow *shadow* – powder-based colour which gives much softer effects.

making eye make-up safe

Eye infections often crop up because eye make-up develops bacteria after it's opened, and these bacteria cause the infection. To limit the risks:

- stop using eye make-up if your eyes are irritated or infected
- wash your hands before applying eye make-up
- don't share your cosmetics with anyone else, not even your best friend
- don't keep your make-up in hot places (like the glove compartment in your car)

shopping for eye make-up

Before you head for the shops or flash your cash:

1. Decide when and where you are going to wear your eye make-up. Natural, muted eyeshadows and pencils are best for daytime definition; but at night you can experiment with more dramatic colours. Just don't overdo the colours.
2. Decide what kind of finish you want – matt, demi-matt or shine. Matt and demi-matt – achieved with powder and solid cream eye shadows – last longest, but demi-matt is kinder on your eyes. Shiny eyeshadow is a directional look best left to make-up artists; it doesn't last and even if you use a fairly standard colour like brown or plum it can make you look like you have got a black eye.
3. Decide how much you want to spend: the conclusion of our tests was that you can get great eye make up from ranges across the board – competitive through to expensive.

... the eye make-up we rate:

Julia Chanel Les 4 Ombres Eyeshadow (£30.50) and Stila Eyeshadow (£12.50): 'I don't think you can beat these two for their colours and durability. Both last so well you never have to worry about them creasing or fading. I think the best eyeliner is Clinique Quick Eyes (£11) – a very soft pencil with a sponge-tip for smudging on the other end. Really quick and easy. And I use Estee Lauder Signature Automatic Pencil for Brows (£15).'

Kate Clinique Touch Tint for Eyes (£12) and Shu Uemura Eyelite Pencil (£10): 'I don't often wear eye make-up, but when I do I use one or both of these. The great thing about the white pencil is that it's mother-of-pearl, so it doesn't just give you flat white colour on your inside lower lash-line. It's far, far softer.'

the 9 best eye cosmetics

the mission to find you the most effective and user-friendly eye make-up on the market.

the criteria our testers judged the eye make-up they tried on their ability to define their eyes and enhance the overall look of their make-up; they reviewed the colours – how good they are, how easy they are to apply and how well they lasted.

Bourjois Suivez Mon Regard Multi-Shimmer Eye Loose Powder £6.50

'I've always been very keen on these,' said Laura (35). 'They're the only eye shadow powders that don't seem to flake and fall off on your face, so they are easier to apply – the applicator brush and screw-off lid help here too, and you don't need to put much of any of the colours on to make an impact.' She also thinks the shadows 'have just the right amount of shimmer – not too disco', and they are perfect for taking on holiday because the shimmer picks up your tan. Party girl Sophie (21) found 'for clubbing they're great. Just the colours I like and they last well too'.

the colours: 14 shades available.

MAC Cream Colour Base £9

A dead cert find in make-up artists' kitbags, these eye shadows were initially developed for professional use only but now we can all buy them. Our testers gave the colours they tried the thumbs up; most commented on how easy they are to apply – 'they don't even need much blending' – and the range of colours. 'There is such a good choice,' said Jane (42), 'and even the classic colours like brown and navy are quite edgy, so you can be quite daring with your eye make-up.' 'Good quality, and they last really well,' said Claire (32). 'I went to the shop to have a browse and thought the assistants were great too. No wonder everyone loves MAC.' Genevieve (35) added, 'They tend to stay where you put them which is always helpful.'

the colours: 18 colours including Fawntastic and Tint, two gorgeous nudes.

Guerlain Divinora Cream To Powder Eye Shadow £13

Gorgeous packaging and yes the price might reflect a chunk of that but we can't get away from the fact that this is a really good eye shadow – our testers have told us so! 'So easy to put on,' said Leah (52). 'It's a cream that turns into a soft powder so you just use a finger to blend it on and it just gives a gentle translucent wash of colour. It's much more flattering than most powder eye shadows too because it doesn't look too matt. In fact it really lifts your eyes and makes them look younger. Lasts well too. Definitely the best eyeshadow I've tried.' What more can we say?

the colours: 10 shades available.

Clinique Touch Tint For Eyes £12

Another popular brand with professionals. This cream-to-powder eyeshadow formula is brilliant and just gives lids a wash of colour and is so idiot-proof to put on you could almost do it without a mirror. The colours are updated seasonally, but the range usually includes some pretty pastels which are great for highlighting your eyes. Lily (51) commented: 'The colour didn't smudge or crease into my eyelids – and that's good going frankly. It's very easy to apply too.' Lisa (37) doesn't usually wear any colour on her eyelids, but she tried these when she went out in the evening and said, 'They add some life to my eyes.' She also said, 'You don't need any level of expertise to apply them.'

the colours: seven in all, including Sable Shimmer, Pink Sheen and Lilac Frost.

Hard Candy Haze Glitter Eye £10.50

We think this is the best glittery eye pencil you can buy. It has a creaminess and softness which is quite unlike any other pencil we have tried – chunky or slim – so you can draw it over your skin without pulling it, which is so important. The makers have not scrimped on the glitter in this product either – you get big chunks of it and the effect is fantastic for a night-time make-up. 'There's a good shot of glitter in each pencil,' said Jane (42), 'so you get a bit of sparkle with every application – not just a bit here and there. And the glittery isn't scratchy either – it can be in make-up.' Liza (30) adores the colours 'especially the pastels because you can't overdo the effects'.

the colours: 11 to choose from (our faves are silver, aubergine and black with gold sparkly bits).

Make Up Forever Colour Liner £8.74

'The best thing about this liner is that it makes drawing a line over your lids so easy. I've always been really nervous of it. I know you can take it off if you boob it, but every time I try and apply liner I start to shake. This liner is so easy to hold though – it's just like a pen, and the colour is so runny it flows really well,' said Annie (26). The line isn't too hard either – often the problem with eyeliner pencils, because the colour is fluid.

the colours: a wide range, including black.

Virgin Vie Eye Definition £6

It is very refreshing to find a decently-priced eye pencil that is soft enough not to drag skin while you apply it – the most important feature for an eye pencil and definitely not the norm as most are too hard. 'It's soft and creamy, a really good value eye pencil,' said Joy (63). And Anne (42) thought it 'gave lovely lasting colour'.

the colours: six colours – Walnut Whip is great for everyday, Storm Cloud is a more steely grey.

Origins Just Browzing £9

Most eyebrow cosmetics either add colour to your brows or fix the hairs in place; this one does both. Shaped like a densely-bristled mascara brush, it dispenses a subtle coating on the hairs and as you apply it, pushes them upwards – which really 'opens' up your eyes – and fixes them in place. 'The colour doesn't go on thickly like with mascara,' wrote Lorna (28), 'and the tone I used – soft black – was so soft you don't end up with Thunderbirds' eyebrows, which is surprisingly easy to do.'

the colours: available in four – blonde, auburn, brown and black.

I.D Bare Escentuals The Perfect Brows £26

An essential kit for the dedicated brow-perfector! The package includes a pot of colour (there are four to choose from covering all tones) with a cleverly-designed angled brow brush and a Brow Finishing Gel to fix the colour and keep it in place. 'The powder is excellent quality and it doesn't spill over onto the rest of your face as you might expect,' said Sarah (23). 'But it is important to follow the instructions – and they are very clear.' You have to swirl the powder around its pot with the brush, tap off the excess and apply it – with feathery strokes – to fill in the gaps between your hairs. Then you set the effects with the gel.

the colours: four in each kit.

mascaras

It never ends does it? The eternal quest for the best mascara in the world. You want volume, you want length, you want curl – you might even want mascara to condition your lashes – but have you ever found one that you are satisfied with?

Very few of us ever buy the same mascara more than twice. Why would we? There are so many of them, each offering better results than the next – it must be a nightmare being a make-up house and trying to get consumers to come back and buy your mascara time and time again. But mascara is mascara – the only cosmetic most women would take to a desert island because it makes such a big impact on your face when you put it on – and so the search for The Perfect Mascara is an ongoing sport.

What do we look for in a mascara? Julia likes chunky lashes and putting on lots of layers. Kate likes a thick, densely bristled brush on a short handle, and thick mascara which beefs up her lashes. She doesn't even mind the odd clump as long as her lashes look thicker. And most of our testers said their dream mascara was one that didn't clump or end up halfway down their faces two hours after putting it on, but that could be removed quite easily when they wanted it to be. Pretty reasonable requests we think.

Whatever you want from mascara – be it fat lashes, thin ones or Twiggy-like curls – our pick of the crop will narrow the search down for you. For this time, anyway.

what makes a good mascara?

- it should last all day without flaking or smudging under your eyes.
- it should not dry up quickly in its tube (a lot do – usually those with thicker brushes that need tubes with bigger openings which let in more air). If it does go dry when it's only a week old you should take it back to the shop.
- it should coat your lashes evenly without leaving clumps on them or sticking them together – but you need to apply it slowly to guarantee this.

how to have clump-free lashes

The reason most of us end up with clogged lashes is because we put mascara on too quickly – it's not always the fault of your mascara. This is how you should do it:

1. Apply a layer of mascara to upper and lower lashes.
2. Wait for at least ten seconds to allow it to dry.
3. Apply a second layer to upper lashes.
4. Need more? Wait for a short time again and apply another coat.
5. If you botch it, wet a cotton Q-tip (saliva is better than water because it's thicker and lifts make-up off your skin more easily) and roll it over your skin.

waterproof or water-soluble?

Waterproof mascara is great if you going on holiday and want to look good on water-skis – and several people who took part in our survey said their dream mascara is a waterproof one which is easy to remove. A lot of us go for waterproof mascaras because we assume that because they can stand up to water they will automatically last longer. It is a clever psychological marketing tactic, but not necessarily true. And anyway, waterproof mascaras that *are* more resilient are trickier to get off, so not ideal for everyday wear because the last thing the skin near your eyes needs is to be rubbed and tugged on a daily basis. Plus, although it can stand up to water, waterproof mascara can still break down and smudge when it comes into contact with oil from your skin or moisturiser. Our advice is to go for ordinary water-soluble ones or have your lashes dyed.

it's just an illusion

Light-reflective particles are now being put into mascaras as well as foundations and concealers to enhance the length, condition and width of your lashes. As with other cosmetics, the particles bounce light off the surface of your lashes in a flattering way, making them look fatter, longer and glossier. Find out which light-reflective mascaras came out top in our road test (see pages 154–156).

coloured mascara: a good thing – or ghastly?

Definitely *good* – on the right faces:

- Khaki and emerald suits redheads with fair skin, brown eyes and olive skin
- Plum and purple make blue eyes look like aquamarines
- Grey looks great with fair and yellow-based skin tones, and all eye colours
- Gold, silver and bronze mascaras look wonderful against dark skins and brown or green eyes
- Red (yes, really) and deep pink looks amazing with dark hair, olive skin and brown eyes. Try it
- White, baby pink and baby blue look good on *no one*, trust us.

‘ever wondered who wears burgundy and plum mascara? If you have got blue eyes you should be! Deep plum and purple mascaras make them look like aquamarines – and make the whites look as bright as Daz’

how to stop mascara drying out

- don't pump the brush in and out of the tube to try and get more mascara on the brush – it will just pump more air in there and make mascara dry up faster.
- don't buy a mascara which comes in a fat tube or with a fat brush unless, like Kate, you are prepared to buy a new one frequently: wide-bristled brushes need a wider tube opening which allows more drying air inside.

never

- put your mascara on when you are mobile – either on public transport or driving (even when you stop at the traffic lights) – even if you are disastrously late for a date.
- wear royal blue mascara (especially with matching eyeliner); it's *so* Eighties.
- go to bed in your mascara – we have all done it (and discovered that it looks strangely good in the morning), but it does your eyes (and the skin around them) no favours. A couple of our testers said that their dream beauty product would be a mascara they could sleep in (ideally by dyeing rather than coating your lashes). This doesn't exist now, but probably will do in the near future.

shopping for mascara

Before you head for the shops or flash your cash:

1. Decide on the colour you want – it's easy to go for black or brown, but colours like plum and grey can do as much, if not more, for your eyes, so experiment.
2. Look at the brush and wands – if you like a thick brush, it's very disappointing to get home and find the one you have bought has a brush with about five bristles in it. You need to work out whether the handle length suits you too, and you will only deduce this by trying the mascara.
3. Decide how much you want to spend: apart from a mid-range mascara by Eyeko, our testers discovered that the best performers came from the cheap and expensive ends of the market – it was half and half.

... mascaras we rate:

Julia Max Factor 2000 Calorie Mascara (£7): 'It lets me build-up layers and thickens my lashes wonderfully. For the price I'm getting a good quality mascara.'

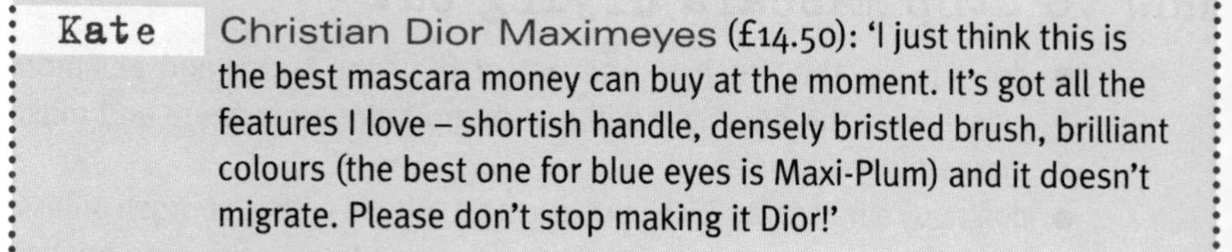

Kate Christian Dior Maximeyes (£14.50): 'I just think this is the best mascara money can buy at the moment. It's got all the features I love – shortish handle, densely bristled brush, brilliant colours (the best one for blue eyes is Maxi-Plum) and it doesn't migrate. Please don't stop making it Dior!'

the 8 best mascaras

the mission to find you the most effective and user-friendly mascaras on the market.

the criteria our testers judged the mascaras they tried on their ability to enhance their eyelashes – without sticking them together in clumps, leaving lumps of hardened mascara on them or flaking off and leaving fibres around their eyes – and make them look longer, curlier, thicker and more lustrous (but not necessarily all at the same time). They also tested mascaras for their consistency, ease of application and removal, and value for money.

Max Factor More Lashes £7.95

From a company who make cosmetics for movie make-up artists (so clearly know what they are doing) – this one got the thumbs up from several testers. 'No clumping or smudging,' wrote Pamela (62), 'in fact I think this is the best mascara I've used.' Clare (29) said, 'It works in a way that I expect mascara to work: it goes on easily (I like to layer it on but you could leave it at a few layers), it lasts extremely well and only came off when I took it off. Really, REALLY good.'

the colours: black, black-brown, brown and navy

Eyeko Mascara £11.50

We wanted to know whether this cult make-up brand sold credible cosmetics and our testers told us: 'Mascara is really important to me because I only ever wear that and a bit of lipgloss, if that,' said Laura (35). 'And you sent me this brilliant mascara! It's so good – I have gorgeous long and luscious lashes. Thanks!' Eyeko Mascara doesn't contain fibres, mineral oil or lanolin – so it could be a good buy for someone who has sensitivity issues with these ingredients. You can use it as eyeliner too by dipping a brush into its air-free (so non-mascara drying) 'toothpaste' tube. Ingenious.

the colours: only black

Almay Double Lash Mascara

£5.99

This mascara was described as a miracle by three of our testers. Kate (42) – who said she has never found a mascara she really likes or bought one twice – gave it ten out of ten. She said, 'It has a short wand, so I thought so far so good when I tested it for the first time, as it was easy to apply. It made my lashes look seriously thick, and it didn't travel. I've got no complaints!' The mascara's lash-thickening powers are put down to a 'quick coat' brush that separates the lashes as you apply it.

the colours: dark brown, black-brown and black-is-black

Collection 2000 Lash Defining Mascara

£2.45

The best cheapie, and hard proof that a good mascara need not be expensive – or even cost you more than a fiver. 'This mascara works so hard,' said Anna (33). 'Some mascaras work well a couple of times and then seem to give up. I've used it everyday since you sent it to me and it's still going – three months later.' Louise (32) thought it performed too: 'It separated and defined my lashes beautifully,' she said, 'I had no clumps either.' The formula contains conditioning agents like provitamin B5.

the colours: only black

Astor Calligraphy Length & Separation Comb Mascara

£7.49

Not your usual method of application – because instead of a brush on a wand you get a comb which feels odd at first, but turns out to be effective because it allows you to get mascara right down to the roots. Deirdre (58) doesn't bother with mascara: 'My lashes are short and dead straight, and none of them ever seem to give enough oomph to make it worthwhile,' she said when we asked her to try this for us. The comb did the trick though because she sent her questionnaire back with a ten out of ten for this one. 'Because you can get the colour right down the lashes it gives them a lift from the base which really makes them look longer and less stick-like,' Deirdre said. 'It did what it said it would do and it met your criteria completely.'

the colours: black and brown

Estée Lauder Magnascopic Maximum Volume Mascara

£15

Dede (48) – a self-confessed mascara-holic – was one of the people who tried this light-reflective mascara and gave it full marks: 'I thought I knew exactly which mascaras were worth buying and which weren't,' she said. 'And when this turned up in the post I thought you had sent me a gimmick to be honest, and an expensive one at that. But I was amazed because it made my lashes look thicker and longer, and I only put on a couple of coats. I can't believe it's taken till now to find it.'

the colours: black, brown, purple and blue

Lancôme Flextencils £16

Lancome are pioneers in the field of mascaras. They are always inventing new ones, and – from the comments we got in our survey – we know they have a faithful following. We got two testers who had not used a Lancome mascara before to try this one for us and the results were both very positive: Lauren (34) said, 'It felt creamy to apply – very smooth application, and it gave my lashes a defined curl.' Genevieve (35) loved the consistency too, and she said 'It stood up to a lot – I wore it in the gym and the rain and it still stayed on, so you can't fault its ability not to smudge.' The mascara includes a patented property called PowerSHAPE – a complex of olive oil, vegetable wax and a silicone coating agent – which enhances lash length and curl.

the colours: black, brown, blue, green and violet

Guerlain Divinora Lengthening & Curving Mascara £14.50

Libby (32) was one of three testers who tried this light-reflective mascara and gave it full marks despite the fact that she thought the wand was a bit long to get the brush close enough to her lash-line. 'My lashes definitely looked longer, which is exactly what I like – I prefer that to chunkier – and they seemed to curl more. The weird thing is though I could swear it works better when you apply less of it – is that possible? Which has to be a real bonus.' It would make sense that this mascara gives better results when used sparingly because of its light-reflective element: it covers lashes in a film which gives them sweeping curl and colour without thickening.

the colours: black, brown, blue and violet

lip colour

For every hundred women who say that mascara would be one of their desert island staples, there are more who would not be parted from their lipsticks or glosses.

We all love lip colour. It finishes your make-up; and it's the quickest way to brighten up your face and make yourself look a bit 'together' – even if you aren't wearing any other make-up. Lipstick gives your face vitality and colour.

There are hundreds of different types of lip cosmetics – lipsticks, lipglosses, tinted balms and fluids; and within those groups there are many different textures and colours too, which can vary greatly even in the same make-up line. Some lip colours are creamy, others dry, greasy, shiny or flat-matt. Some glide evenly over your lips and melt after five minutes: others smear or go on stickily and last for hours.

Finding one that you like is a question of trial and error, so lip stick is a bit like mascara in this sense – you always feel you can get a better one.

Which is quite possible, especially if you have not tried any of our top ten lip colours. Read on if you want to know how good lip colour can be.

what makes good lip colour? (in order of importance)

1. **durability** – despite the fact that there are so many different types of lip colour, the one common virtue they should all share is long life. It doesn't matter whether it's lipstick, gloss, tinted balm, liquid 'lipstick' or any other kind of lip colour, the one thing we all want is for it to stay on for as long as possible.
2. **colour** – it might sound like we are stating the obvious here, but we want good quality colour too. The pigment must spread well (this is especially important when it's a darker colour) so the colour goes on evenly all over your lips.
3. **application** – lip colour must be easy to apply. Tinted balms should never be solid, glosses should glide easily over lips on a fingertip, and lipsticks should be resilient enough to smooth colour on our lips without breaking in half.

never

- wear glittery lip colour (especially if you are serious about your career) unless you are under 16 or going to a fancy dress party; it is very unflattering and very different to lightly shimmering gloss
- use a lip pencil that is darker than your lipstick or gloss – it looks really, really awful
- wear dark matt lip colour if you have got thin lips – it will make them look much thinner
- wear pale iridescent lipstick – it makes your lips look as if they have got frostbite and you will look like an extra from *Heartbeat*

always

- blot lipstick with a tissue or bit of loo paper when you have applied it, then apply a second layer – this trick doubles its lifespan
- apply lipstick and gloss with a brush – you get better accuracy – and, for some reason we haven't yet got to the bottom of, it makes lip colour last longer
- stroke a cotton Q-tip around your lip-line to soften the line of your lipstick

do you need a lip pencil?

Not that long ago it was unthinkable to apply lipstick or gloss without first lining your lips in a matching pencil. This was a dire make-up moment because the lipstick invariably wore off leaving you with a mouth ringed in liner (not a good look) – the reason lip pencils went out of favour again. It must be said, however, that if it's applied properly (and you use a colour that matches your lips – not your lipstick), lipliner does go a long way to help lip colour stay on. If you are still wearing it – and finding that it outlives your lip colour – try this:

1. Trace around your lips (excluding the bow) lightly with the pencil then use it to shade in half of your upper and lower lips.
2. Apply a coat of lipstick or gloss and blot the whole lot with a tissue.
3. Trace around the outside of your lips with a damp Q-tip to soften the line – it can look very hard.
4. Apply a second coat of lipstick or gloss and blot again.

beauty scoop highly commends:

- MAC Spice Lip Pencil (£9): we still think this is one of the best lipliners you can buy (if not *the* best); it is a perfect cinnamon-flesh tone and genuinely suits every skin colour.

can you wear red lipstick?

We can't count the times we have heard people say they can't wear red lip colour. They insist it either looks brassy on them because they are

beauty scoop highly commends:

- best for fair skins and blonde hair: Laura Mercier Geranium Lip Kiss (£15) is very transparent – more like a tinted balm disguised as a lipstick, and the colour is so soft you could put it on without looking, but it's *still* a true red.
- best for fair and yellow-based complexions and dark hair: MAC Liza Red Lipstick (£11) is named after Liza Minnelli. Say no more.
- best for dark skins and hair: Benefit Such A Red Marvelous Lips (£11.50) is a pure, deep red – only *you* can pull it off!

very fair or makes them look like a china doll. But we think everyone should have some red lip colour in their make-up bag – it's so glam and grown-up. Red lip colour is the little black dress of the make-up world – and we swear there is one out there for *everyone*, no matter what your colouring. It's just a question of finding the right shade, consistency and finish.

shopping for lip cosmetics

Before you head for the shops or flash your cash:

1. Work out which tones you look best in – it could be blue-based pinks or more coral or yellow tones – and when you are at the counter, try lip-colours on the inside of your wrist to see if the colour suits your skin.
2. Decide what finish you want. Lipsticks come in matt, shine or satin (halfway between matt and shine); lipglosses are obviously glossy; liquid lipsticks (applied on a wand) can be glossy or matt, and balms are shiny but not as glassy as gloss. Satin and slightly sparkling or light-reflective lip colours are the most flattering on most lips – matt can be very ageing.
3. Decide when you are going to wear it – to work, at weekends or in the evening? Natural colours make you look groomed but not over-made-up in the day; and we recommend red or darker colours like plum in the evening.
4. Decide how much you want to spend: our testers found that lipsticks and glosses across the board – from cheap to expensive – performed well.

... the lip cosmetics we rate:

Julia MAC Lipstick (£11): 'I've always loved MAC lipsticks – especially the shade Twig. They have got brilliant lasting power and the colours are great. Laura Mercier Bare Lips and Dusty Rose Lip colours (£14) are always in my handbag.'

Kate Bobbi Brown SPF15 Lip Shine (£13): 'Probably my number one lipstick – I love every shade (especially Rouge Brilliant) and its slim-line shape. I think Revlon LipGlide Color Gloss (£7.49) has the best lip colour finish – it's somewhere between satin lipstick and gloss – quite unique.'

the best lip colours

the mission: to find you the most effective and user-friendly lipsticks and glosses on the market.

the criteria our testers judged the lip colours they tried on their colour depth, appeal and trueness, staying-power, finish – if matt, they had to be non-shiny without bobbling, if satin they could not be too shiny, and if shiny not too slippery or glassy (yes, we are hard task masters!) The lip colours' application and value for money were reviewed too, and to bring you the absolute crème de la crème of glosses, our testers looked for special individual qualities in each.

the 5 best lipsticks

Chanel Rouge A Levres Hydrabase £14

For a lipstick that was launched in 1972 this is quite an accolade. It was originally developed to provide lips with colour, as well as moisturising and protecting them – quite a pioneering idea 30 years ago. It still has these qualities and is now available in iridescent and metallic variations, and satin or matt finishes, too. 'Great colours and –I've got to say it – stylish packaging, there's nothing like that solid "click" when the lip goes back on,' says Laura (35). 'I absolutely love Chanel lipsticks,' said Katie (39). 'You can't get better colour depth, and the texture is so wonderfully creamy. It has to be the best you can buy.'

the colours: a huge colour range which is constantly under review.

Max Factor Lipfinity £9.99

Most of the make-up houses went through a phase of trying to bring us longer-lasting lipsticks – some of them still are. But pretty much all of them were horribly drying on your lips because they had such a high density of pigment in them, so they died a fast death. This one has lasted the course because it works best. 'It feels a bit dry when the lip paint dried, but once you've got the moisturising top coat on your lips feel supple,' said Sandra (41). 'I'm keeping it.' Clare (41) said, 'It lasts so well but I had to keep stopping myself from applying more gloss because I assumed I needed it.' And Caroline (38) added, 'The first time I tried it, it did what it claimed and lasted all day – through coffee and ciggie breaks and right up until I had a Chinese takeaway that night.'

the colours: 21 – plus two top coat shades.

Rimmel Lasting Finish Lipstick £3.99

A good creamy textured lipstick – at a brilliant price. Rimmel updated the formula recently to give it added shine and greater endurance; it now promises to stay on (depending on what you are doing) for seven hours. 'A good moisturising lipstick that happens to last well – as long as it claims, if not longer – and a fantastic price,' said Hannah (31). 'I've always liked Rimmel cosmetics,' said Magda (29), 'they are a good price, the colours are great and this is a superb lipstick. Why would you spend more on another?'

`the colours:` 26 in the range.

Clarins Le Rouge £13

This is a classic Clarins' lipstick – longlasting, creamy and comfortable to wear. There is nothing fussy or particularly unusual about it; it uses a polymer resin to preserve the colour pigments, and this is what gives it such intense lasting colour. Joan (40), one of the testers who love this lipstick, said it was her 'ideal lipstick', and gave her 'a good strong colour without being drying on my lips'.

`the colours:` nearly 40 shades in the range.

RMK Irresistible Lips £15

'Despite its sheer texture the staying-power of this lipstick is excellent and I found it very comfortable to wear,' said Joy (63). 'I've never heard of the brand before but I'm really impressed.' The formula comes in two variations – sheer colour or more intense with a matt finish, and the lipsticks are presented in typically Japanese simple silver containers. 'The pink shade I tried is heavenly,' said Lou (68). 'My only problem is the Japanese writing on the packaging. What does it mean?'

`the colours:` about 45 – and growing.

the 8 best lipglosses

best lip-plumper

Ultima II Extraordinaire Volumizing Lip Gloss £13.95

We remember when these were first launched: everyone suddenly cottoned-on to how good they were and rushed off to stock up on them. They are still as popular now because the formula – a hydro lip-volumising complex of super-moisturising molecules – is still unrivalled in its ability to make lips look fuller. 'The gloss is quite slippery if you know what I mean,' said Eve (37), 'but the result is amazing – is it the shimmer in it that makes my lips look more pouty?'

the colours: six shades, including the most natural – Bare Boost.

best staying power

Cosmetics A La Carte Lip Gloss £17

'I wouldn't fancy kissing anyone wearing this,' wrote Tessa (35). 'I think we would end up glued together. The gloss is that clingy – which is a good thing I suppose – and it also stains your lips a bit which helps the colour to stay put. I love the colours too.' The most popular shades are Candy, a soft pink, Vamp and a clear gloss called Lip Glass which can be worn on its own or over lipstick.

the colours: so many it is almost impossible to count, but we think two of the most wearable are Blush and Gold.

best shine

Bourjois Effet 3D High Shine £6.75

Bourjois' beauty scientists have added a faint pearlised element to these glosses which give them a 3D effect – and this boosts their shine and gives the colours extra depth. It is a very popular gloss with celebrities because it gives lips a high shine without being too glassy – effects which work really well on TV. 'I like the fact it gives your lips a hint of colour – not too full-on solid colour – which can look too much for a gloss,' said Sally (22). 'And the colours are really fashionable. It's such a great brand.'

the colours: tbc

best application

Stila Lip Glaze £18

Our testers particularly liked the click-and-lick pen-like applicator of this lipgloss – you just have twist one end for it to dispense the right amount of gloss. 'It does work well – so often when cosmetics companies try to give us new-fangled things they end up being gimmicky and break down,' said Susie (31). 'But this keeps going. I also love the flavours, especially melon – I wore it all summer.' Its pretty range of sheer colours is constantly updated; we think this is the perfect gloss to take on holiday.

the colours: 15 colours – the most wearable being the natural nude, Cinnamon.

best packaging

Chanel Levres Scintillantes Glossimer £13

Lots of those who took part in our survey said that packaging is very important to them – so don't blame us for adding a 'best packaging' winner to this round-up of the best lipglosses! 'A good amount of stickability on my lips without the feeling that they are glued together,' said Laura (35). The packaging of course is too gorgeous – you won't fail to impress if you pull this out of your handbag. 'They are seriously lovely glosses. Great to look at and just enough colour and shine,' said Laura.

the colours: a range of eight shades.

best value

Collection 2000 Plastique Lipgloss £2.19

Having tried a variety of different lipglosses at all prices, Jane (40) has decided that this brilliantly priced gloss is the best, claiming 'it's a joy to use'. Annie (26) said: 'I really like the glittery clear gloss – I put it over normal lipstick to add a touch of shimmer. And price-wise you can't go wrong.' Our only advice is to try before you buy because the shades tend to be stronger than they look on the shade charts.

the colours: 15 different ones including Pink Berry and Cherry (quite a daring red).

best for hip chicks

Pixi Lip Gloss £12

The Pixi beauty boutique is like the sweetest candy shop in London – the choice of cosmetics leaves you quite literally dazed. They are well known for their lipgloss formulas, but we (and our testers) think this one is the best: 'The colours are the best in this range. I've probably got half of them in my make-up bag,' said Tania (29). And Harriet (41) goes for the taste of the gloss – a sort of caramel-vanillary or peppermint flavour. 'It just never stays on for very long as it tastes too divine,' she said.

the colours: we gave up counting (but there are about 24).

best flavour

Lancôme Juicy Tubes £11.50

Oh boy, does everyone love these Juicy Tubes – or what? Lancôme say they sell one of them every 75 seconds and the testers we introduced to them went mad over them. 'Forget mascara, I can't leave home without this,' said Emma (44). 'I'd take it to my desert island.' 'These are the best lipglosses around,' said Mandy (33). And 'I wouldn't use any other now. The gloss is great and it tastes yummy,' said Caroline (42). Do we need to say anymore?!

the colours: over a dozen, including Rose Glacé and Sorbet. Yum.

face powders

Powder is an underrated cosmetic. You rarely read about it – mainly because it stops your face from looking shiny, and shiny – sorry, *glowing* – skin looks younger and healthier than a powdery one. Everyone over the age of 16 wants their complexion to have a satin or demi-matt (halfway between shiny and matt) finish now – and for a good reason: it is ten times more flattering than a matt finish, which can make your face look flat, old and more lined.

'powders with a UV filter are a good thing, but it is worth bearing in mind that they tend to be a bit thicker than those that don't contain sunscreens'

Which doesn't leave powder with much of a role – except to blot the oil off your nose (no one wants a shiny nose) or dust down excessive shine in the day. Or does it?

Read on and you will find out how the right powder, used the right way, can actually be as powerful as foundation at enhancing and maximising your skin.

how powder has changed

You can understand why people went off powder – until very recently it did nothing but turn your face into a flat pancake. But it has changed, believe us! This is how:

1. Most powders are much more finely milled than they were even ten years ago (Prescriptives' Magic Illuminating Powder needs to be felt to be believed), which means they give a much sheerer finish – so much so that many are imperceptible.
2. Some powders contain light-reflectors, so far from giving you a flat, matt face they actually make your skin glow in the same way as some clever foundations can.
3. Powders may also contain sunscreens – clever, especially for people who don't want to wear face cream or foundation with chemical sun filters in them.
4. A few powders are even clever enough to moisturise your skin and keep it supple, so you don't get that horrible dry, tight and powdery look anymore.

what about talc in powders – is it a friend or foe?

Something else that put people off face powder is the ingredient talc – which has had a very bad press over the years after some studies found that when it is used in pure and large amounts as talcum powder it may have sinister health implications. Apart from the fact that there needs to be more research done on this, face powder includes nothing like the concentration of talc as regular talcum powder does. The concern about talc is not actually about its use in make-up, so there is no reason to avoid cosmetics that contain it.

how to get the right shade of powder

Our tips on choosing the right colour are:

1. Powder should match the colour of your skin and your foundation – not change either. So test it the same way you would foundation – on your face (ideally with a sample you can try at home in natural light) and with your foundation.
2. Avoid powders with a white (that doesn't mean mother-of-pearl), orange, pink or coral hue; they will make you look a strange colour or over made-up.
3. If in doubt go for translucent – but remember to try it before buying it because even translucent powder has a hint of colour in it.

how to apply powder

1. Powder should go on over foundation or directly onto bare skin – and only to the areas you need it. These are usually your T-zone – forehead, cheeks and chin – areas which have a greater density of sebaceous glands so are oilier and shinier.
2. Some loose powders come with a brush, but as well as being wasteful (because you lose half the powder when you start dusting it over your face) brushes don't allow you to use powder to 'fix' skin or foundation because you can't make it adhere properly. Use a non-fluffy powder pad or latex sponge (Kate thinks this is the best applicator because it allows you to press powder into your skin) and after picking powder up on it shake some back into the pot so you don't apply too much.
3. After you have applied powder, skim over your face with a cottonwool bud to take off any excess.

'the difference between pressed powder and loose? Pressed powder is heavier and has added waxes or emollients in it to keep it solid. It is also less messy'

avoid

- Powdering over a matt foundation – even on your nose (unless you have severely oily skin): it will make you look like a shriveled up old lizard.
- Layering on powder: the less you build up on your face the less made-up you will appear (the aim for so many of us), and over-powdering makes your face look dull and dry, especially if you have dry skin already or a darker skin tone.
- Applying powder too many times during the day. A good powder should stay put so that you only have to retouch it a couple of times a day. However clever powder has got, it can very quickly look heavy and thick if you are not careful.
- Wearing powder with gold sparkly bits in it. This is a very different thing to light-reflective particles (which you can't see anyway), and looks extremely naff unless you have a light tan and the effects are very subtle. You have been warned!

shopping for powder

Before you head for the shops or flash your cash:

1. Decide whether you want a compact (best for carrying around with you to do re-touches) or a loose one.
2. Work out which shade of powder will suit you – or, to be on the safe side, decide to go for a translucent one.
3. Decide how much you want to spend: our testers found that powders in the mid to premium range brands performed best.

... powders we rate:

Julia Benefit Dandelion (£22 for 10gm): 'I love everything about this powder – the colour, the fineness of the powder and (dare I say it) the packaging.'

Kate Prescriptives Magic Illuminating Powder (£29 for 35gm): 'I don't use powder very often and when I do I always wear it on its own – not over foundation – and I think this does the job best. I just can't see how you can better this powder.'

the 5 best face powders

the mission: to find you the most effective and user-friendly face powders on the market.

the criteria our testers judged the powders they tried on their ability to enhance their skin – not just zap shine – preserve their make-up and keep it looking fresh. They also reviewed powders for ease of application, colour and durability.

Benefit Dandelion
£22 for 10gm

A cult powder – it is used by celebrities, make-up artists and beauty journalists because it is like an instant pick-me-up for your skin. 'I wasn't quite sure how to use it at first,' said Jo (33), 'it doesn't look like an ordinary powder and I have to say that for me its packaging worked against it because it's so good I couldn't imagine that the powder would be up to much! It *so is* though. It really lifts your face and gets rid of that grey look, that's the best way to describe its effect. I absolutely love it.'

the science bit: a fine blend of pink and mauve particles – with a subtle smattering of gold flecks – that have an instant brightening effect on tanned skin.

Prescriptives Magic Illuminating Powder
£25 for 28gm

A unique face powder – no other feels like this to touch, it has the most extraordinary texture. Judy (57) was quite taken aback by it. She said, 'It feels almost damp because it's so soft – it's really weird. Then you put it on and it makes your skin look and feel so soft and fresh. It is a powder, but it's not – it's out of this world. I wore it with foundation and without – for about the first time in thirty years – and was more than happy with the results. It's a great find and I would never have tried it otherwise. I'm hooked.'

the science bit: a state-of-the-art light-reflective powder, it uses soft optics to diffuse light and minimise fine lines, and enhances the effects of your foundation.

Ultima II Extraordinaire Silk Touch Pressed Powder
£18.50 for 10gm

'Great looking compact,' said Hilly (27), 'and that's the important thing with portable powder I think. It's a lovely shiny silver one, very chic.' Looks aren't all though: 'It's pleasantly lightweight, which came as a bit of a surprise,' Hilly said, 'because I always assume powder will be cakey. And it doesn't matter how often you put it on you don't get that horrible crusty build-up. It's got a nice fluffy puff too; it's good value.'

the science bit: contains a sunscreen, antioxidant vitamins A, C and E, and oil blotters to limit shine breakthrough. Available in three shades.

Bourjois Libre Comme L'Air

£9.95 for 6gm

A loose powder packaged in a portable stick-like tube (how ingenious is that?) with a neat little brush applicator – so it's an all in one. 'The only drawback I had with it is that I found the brush a bit hard at first,' said Sue (51); 'other than that I could not fault it.' Anne (26) was impressed too: 'The shade I used is near-perfect for my colouring and the packaging is incredibly convenient. No mess and no waste. Brilliant!'

the science bit: contains nylon powder to soak up excess oil and kaolin powder to give skin a soft matt finish. Available in four shades.

Givenchy Prisme Again! Visage

£22 for 10gm

Recently reinvented, this powder has been upgraded to compete with the leaders in the field and got good reviews from our testers. It is still a prism powder – incorporating a quartet of pressed powders in varying pastel shades which, when mixed with the brush as you apply it, help to make the powder match your skin colour more closely. It also boosts radiance because it has a slight iridescence to it and gives a matt finish. Those who have tried it include Margaret (62) who said: 'It works so well, you can't see it and it doesn't clog up your skin or feel heavy. I didn't feel like it had put years on me – a lot of powders do you know!'

the science bit: the powder contains treatment ingredients like dog rose extract – an emollient – and the antioxidant gingko biloba. Available in six colourways.

nail colours

Ever since Uma Thurman appeared in *Pulp Fiction* wearing Chanel's Rouge Noir nail polish in 1999 coloured lacquer has never gone back out of fashion. It was as if a light had pinged on and everyone suddenly realised that nail polish isn't just something you only wear when you are dressed-up and going out; it's as much an everyday cosmetic as mascara, especially if you want to look polished.

Having said that we think you need to be quite discerning about the colours you wear. Certain varnishes are better off on children's fingernails than adults. Nail polishes with big glittery bits in them, a matt finish and in colours like blue and green have no place on your bathroom shelf – let alone your fingernails – they are horrible!

'personally, we hate false nails – they look tacky (especially if they are painted with glittery polish). Just don't go there'

In our survey, a lot of testers said that they rarely spent much on nail polish – stocking up on the cheapie brands and using them once or twice like gimmicks – but they loved the idea of owning a varnish by Chanel or a similar upmarket brand.

So the challenge here is to find three or four polishes that you would be happy to wear with jeans, a work suit and after-six dress: a soft beige perhaps, a clear varnish, a deep red and a modern brown-based pink – and you want them all to be as hard-wearing (that means last longer than a day before chipping) and glossy as possible.

Look no further: thanks to our intrepid testers we have found what we (and they) believe to be the best nail polishes money can buy.

what makes a good nail varnish? (in order of importance)

1. **colour** – if you love it and it suits your skin tone you will wear the varnish again and again no matter how difficult it is to apply or how long it lasts.
2. **texture & finish** – a decent varnish should not be too runny or too thick (some thicken over time and the only solution is to bin them and buy another), and should have a really glossy finish (unless it says it's matt).
3. **drying time** – the quicker the better; but it's always best to leave freshly-painted nails for at least an hour before you start rummaging around in your handbag, getting dressed or having a bath.
4. **durability** – most varnishes don't last longer than a few days before they start to look tired enough to be redone; but the best last for at least a week.
5. **application** – the brush should be medium thickness, the handle should be easy to grip and on the long side of stubby (but not so long that you can't get close enough to your nail when applying the varnish.

always

- remove all traces of moisturiser from your nails before you apply varnish: moisturising ingredients stop varnish adhering to them
- apply polish in layers allowing each one to dry before applying the next
- allow lots of time for nail varnish to dry – longer than you think: you don't want to spend ages applying it only to have to start again because it's scuffed or smudged. Running a gentle stream of cold water over your nails – or dipping them in cold cooking oil – can help varnish to dry quicker. You can also buy quick-dry sprays, top coats and oils, but make sure they don't have alcohol in them as this will make the varnish peel off or chip faster

never

- dry nail polish with a hairdryer or any other heat source: heat makes the colour expand and lift away from your nails
- soak your nails in hot, soapy water for longer than a few minutes to soften the cuticles; it damages them
- do the washing up without rubber gloves on: detergent and hot water are a killer combo for nails

shopping for nail varnishes?

Before you head for the shops or flash your cash:

1. Decide when – and with what – you are going to wear your nail polish: to work or to a party? Not all colours work in both situations or with all clothes.
2. Sample the varnish – the colour usually looks different on your nails to how it does in the bottle and it may be more transparent than you would like.
3. Decide how much you are going to spend: our testers found that, on the whole, the cheaper nail polishes performed better than the expensive ones, and several said they would not dream of spending more than a tenner on varnish. Unless it happened to be by Chanel...

'to make fat fingers appear slimmer, paint a single stripe down the centre of your nails with a dark polish'

... nail varnishes we rate:

Julia 'Pass! I don't wear it.'

Kate Nails Inc Nail Polish (£8.50 for 8ml) – they are the glossiest, seem to be the most durable and come in a brilliant range of colours. I've got through two or three bottles of their Tate shade, it's a perfect blue-red.'

the 5 best nail polishes

the mission: to find you the most effective and user-friendly nail polishes on the market.

the criteria our testers judged the nail polishes they tried on their colour – its depth, wearability and durability – the speed with which it chipped or faded, gloss, ease of application (that included the length and thickness of the brush), drying time, value for money and whether it lived up to its claims.

Jessica Custom Nail Colour £7.15 for 14.8ml

Not many of our testers had heard of this brand, but those who had – and had a Jessica manicure or pedicure (professional manicurists rave about this range) – rated the nail care and polishes very highly. 'It's the only polish I've ever come across that truly doesn't chip after 48 hours,' said Pauline (47). And Jackie (34) backed that up by writing 'Brilliant! It stayed on and it didn't chip until I took it off five days later. I think that's very good going.' Caroline (38) said she thought the best thing about this polish was its application: 'You can tell it's good quality because you only have to put one coat on for it to look perfect.'

Rimmel 60 Seconds Nail Polish £2.89 for 8ml

Out of all the quick speed dry polishes this came out way above everything else in our survey – partly because it dries hard quickly and comes in an extensive range of colours. Faye (58) commented: 'It doesn't strictly dry hard in 60 seconds – I can't honestly say that. But it is still very quick, much more so than any other polish I've used, and I did put on two coats, not one. I'd say it dried hard enough not to smudge in less than five minutes. Lasted well too.' Catherine (40) was so impressed she told us she is ready to move on from her old favourite: 'I've been a fan of Chanel's nail enamel for years, but I do prefer this and I presume it's a fraction of the cost.' And just to push the message about this polish's performance home, Anne (42) added: 'Perfect coverage in just one coat. It did what it said it would do!'

Revlon Colorstay Overtime Nail Enamel

£6.49 for colour and top coat 10ml each

When we asked our testers to tell us what their favourite nail brand is, Revlon's name came up most often. We got comments like 'the most durable nail polishes', 'they last for ages' and 'in my price league' stood out. This particular polish claims to last a staggering ten days because it has a built-in 'top coat' which acts like a sealant and protects from exterior damage (which makes total sense to us). 'I applied two coats,' said Annalise (25), 'and it didn't chip off.' After testing this varnish for us, Lucy (32) went shopping for more and fell for the colours: 'They're just so many good ones to choose from and they're as good if not better than the pricy ones,' she said.

L'Oréal Ceramide Resist

£4.99 for 9ml

"I've always been a bit anti nail varnish,' said Louise (32), 'because my nails are so thin and flaky and I just think putting colour on them like that is going to make them worse.' We sent her this 'treatment varnish' to try (it contains an ingredient called ceramide R which is said to help strengthen nails) and kept our fingers crossed. She sent her questionnaire back and had written 'unbelievably hardy as a varnish and I've had no breaks or splits while wearing it or since. What's in it?!' Sal (24) added: 'I love the colour I tried – a pinky-beige – which you forget you are wearing, as half the reason I don't wear varnish is because it makes me too aware of my hands.'

Chanel Nail Enamel

£12 for 13ml

As far as many of our testers were concerned you can't better Chanel's nail polishes: 'You've got to admit it IS the best packaging in the world,' said Susie (31), 'it looks so luxurious and chic and that really matters.' We agree! 'As much as I love Chanel make-up it's completely beyond my budget,' said Susie, 'but I will treat myself to the varnish, and it's a good buy. It lasts well, the colours are mouth-watering and the application is the easiest of all varnishes. Perfect size handle, perfect length brush and density of bristles. Chanel have really done their research.' The colour most of our testers have tried (and still wear) is Rouge Noir, the popular black-red. No surprise then that it is still on waiting lists everywhere four years after its launch.

NAIL CARE

The message came across loud and clear in our survey: you *love* coloured varnish (especially plum, beige and mother-of-pearl), but nail care products are not big on your agendas at all (you don't have time) and when you buy nail products you tend to go for the cheaper brands sold in chemists rather than schlep to salons for specialist products.

> 'top manicurist Marian Newman's best low-maintenance tip for nails is to massage a little olive into the cuticles every night to keep them supple and healthy'

We both freely admit to not paying much attention to our nails (Kate is the only one of us who bothers with coloured nail polish), and we were quite surprised to find that most of the people who took part in our survey are as dispassionate about their nails as we are! Either that, or you are confused about the nail care products you need.

So having manicures *is* still a big deal for most of us; despite the pit stop nail bars in department stores around the country and the ongoing use of coloured lacquers, we are not – and probably never will be – anywhere near as nail obsessed as American women.

If you are going to use nail care products, you want them to work fast and effectively; and you only want to be told about products that are essential. So that is what we are doing here. As well as some down-to-earth advice on nail care (some of which might surprise you), you will find out which products our testers gave top marks to.

What you will find out about in this chapter:

- Why you need a base coat if you are wearing coloured nail polish
- The lowdown on 'fast-drying' polish
- Whether there is any point eating raw jelly chunks

nail essentials

Our motto for nails – as with most of beauty – is to keep things as simple as possible. We know from your responses to our survey that nail care products are not a big priority – you don't have the time for regular manicures (either at home or in a salon); so we asked our testers to try products we think should be every woman's nail essentials. This covered nail strengtheners, cuticle moisturisers or softeners, base and top coats (some of which double-up as quick drying overcoats for coloured polish). Find out which ones worked best on the following pages.

an important word about cuticles

Cuticles are probably the only part of our nails that actually benefit from the fact that we are not a nation of manicure addicts, because the best way to keep your nails healthy is to push your cuticles back *as little as you can*. In fact, the less you manipulate and cut them the better. Susan Gerrard of The Natural Nail Company maintains that 'you should never cut cuticles because they grow back quicker, thicker and harder'. Apart from inherited problems and physical trauma (like shutting your fingers in a door or having your toe trodden on by an elephant), damage from over-pushing and over-trimming cuticles is the biggest cause of nail problems and can alter their growth. This might come as a surprise if you have been led to believe that you should regularly push cuticles back – or indeed 'remove' them – as some products claim to do. Cuticles are there for a reason: to protect and seal the live part of your nail beneath the skin. And the most you should do is apply hand cream or softening balm to them whenever you remember to stop them getting dry and flaky.

> 'eat raw jelly chunks because you love them, not because you think the gelatin in them will make your nails stronger: it won't!'

beauty scoop highly commends:

- Sally Hansen 3-in-1 Cuticle Quencher Crème (£6.95 for 19.8ml) – contains nourishing vitamin E and softens up cuticles after one application without making skin or nails greasy.

who needs nail strengthener?

Nails are basically a protective covering of dead cells filled with a thick protein called keratin. They are quite similar in make up to your hair. Some of us are born with naturally thick, hard nails; but most of us have soft nails that flake off easily (except in summer when exposure to the sun and sea often toughens them up) and need to fortify them. Now, here is another little revelation: diligently applying nail care products *does* help to strengthen nails, but it's the physical protective coating they provide that does the trick, not the ingredients. So don't let anyone tell you that you can only have a decent set of nails if you use products with ingredients like calcium or proteins in them – it's simply not true.

is there a nail varnish that 'really does dry quickly'?

A lot of them make this claim but a few live up to it. However, it must be said that the way you apply nail polish is a major factor in its lifespan. It's boring we know, but base and top coats are essential if you want coloured varnish to stay put and not chip – no matter how resilient it claims to be. Base coats prime your nails, make varnish cling on harder and stop it staining your nails; top coats stop varnish from chipping and fading, make it look glossier and the really good ones make it dry faster too.

... nail treatments we rate:

Julia Elizabeth Arden Eight Hour Cream (£13 for 50ml): 'Like most people I don't have time to do my nails and after years of abuse (biting, mostly) I'm the first to admit that they look pretty awful. When they're really bad this faithful balm comes out again – I put it on my cuticles at night and it softens them up. OPI Nail Envy Natural Nail Strengthener (£14.95 for 15ml) is the only product that has ever made a real difference to the strength of my nails.'

Kate Supernail of LA Emergency Stikr (£4.95 for 5gm or £8.95 for 8gm brush-on): 'Essential if your nails constantly break off – even when they're not very long. It's the only nail care product I use.'

the 3 best nail care products

the mission to find you the most effective and user-friendly nail care products on the market.

the criteria our testers judged the nail care products they tried on their ability to strengthen nails and improve their flexibility and appearance; add shine and durability to coloured varnishes; and speed up drying time for varnishes. They also tested nail products for efficacy, value for money and the level of their instructions.

OPI Nail Envy Natural Nail Strengthener — £14.95 for 15ml

This is a great all-round product. Its main aim is to strengthen your nails but it can be also used as a base and/or top coat, so it helps to preserve your nail polish too. Julia bangs on about it being the best thing that has happened to her nails in 39 years all the time, and several of our testers agree with her. Jane (67) had given up trying to find something to make her nails less brittle – she put it down to age, but said that this product 'instantly hardened my nails so they didn't constantly break and split'. Jennifer (30) has weak nails because she is a phantom nail-chewer, but said, 'It works so quickly I managed to resist nibbling my nails while I had it on. It's made a big difference to the length of my nails.' Apply every other day for week, then remove and start the regime again.

the science bit: formulated with hydrolysed wheat protein, which – OPI claim – strengthens nails without making them brittle.

Barielle Natural Nail Camouflage Anti-aging Growth Enhancer — £15 for 14ml

Some of our older testers complained of having very ridged nails, saying they look unsightly, that it is hard to use any kind of polish over them without putting on lots of layers and was there anything they could do about it? We asked some of them to try this product for us. It claims to fill in the ridges – not get rid of them – giving nails a smoother finish. Three of our testers gave it 10/10. 'It's a very pale pinky tone that I thought would look awful on my nails, but it actually gives hardly any colour at all,' wrote Gill (71). 'And it improved the look of my nails straightaway.'

the science bit: contains ingredients that fill in the ridges and a blend of vitamins and vegetable proteins which, it is claimed, stop them getting worse and to protect nails from breaks.

Creative Nail Design Super Shiny High Gloss Top coat

£8.95 for 15ml

We sent out so many top coats for testing we nearly lost count of them, and the verdict on this one was way ahead of any others; it was outstanding. Our testers said it gave bare nails and polishes an incredible shine which seemed to last beyond 24 hours, and it didn't need topping-up – because it had chipped or worn – for periods varying between five to eight days. 'It's a really good protective cover and it gives a very high sheen,' said Joy (63). 'Proof – if it's needed – that the Americans really come up with the best nail products.'

the science bit: the key ingredient is a controversial one – toughening tuolene (see page 187) –which, say Creative Nail Design, is used in 'minimal' amounts.

TOOLS OF THE TRADE

Every so often you pick up some really valuable little beauty gems when you read about the accessories – tweezers, brushes, nail files, that sort of thing – that the experts 'can't live' without. You tear the snippet out of the magazine (sneakily, if you are in the dentist's waiting room) ready to take on your next shopping trip .. and you lose it.

'one of the biggest mistakes we make when blow-drying our hair is to stop (usually because our arms are aching or we are bored) before hair is fully dry – which is why you end up with a frizzy do rather than something more controlled'

So how much more useful would it be to have that information in a book you can keep in your handbag? We thought so.

This section details the best beauty gizmos – from make-up brushes to hairdryers and tweezers – those tools of the trade that the experts swear by because they make such light work of beauty chores such as straightening your hair and plucking your eyebrows. These are the best beauty accessories your money can buy. Trust us: we have seen them in the professionals' kitbags and we have got most of them ourselves.

What you will find out about in this chapter:

- That you don't need eyelash curlers (especially not heated ones) if you have got a decent mascara
- Why a round or straightening brush makes a far better (and less ageing) job of straightening your hair than ceramic irons
- That not all body brushes are the same
- How properly plucked and shaped eyebrows can take years off your face
- How to re-touch your own roots

beauty accessories

By now you will have hopefully got the message that the best beauty regimes are the simplest ones. It makes sense to us that once you have got the basics like foundation and moisturiser sorted you can have fun experimenting with more gimmicky products.

Your beauty basics are fashion's equivalent of a little black dress, white shirt, boot-leg jeans and cashmere sweater: they are the cornerstones of your beauty 'wardrobe'. They are the products and gadgets that you can rely on to deliver the goods (be it to buff your nails or straighten your hair) every time you use them. And they include accessories like a sharp pair of easy-to-grip tweezers, a decent set of make-up brushes and a round brush.

We have both been lucky enough to have worked with lots of make-up and hair professionals in our careers – and so are in a position to find out what they really carry around in their kitbags. And much of what has made it onto *Beauty Scoop*'s best list here has been picked up this way. Some of the stuff might not be what you expect. But the professionals don't always rely on the most technical and swanky-looking gadgets; they hang on to the accessories that deliver the goods every time. Read on to find out what these accessories are.

beauty gadgets everyone should have

- a decent pair of tweezers – sharp and easy to grip
- a durable nail file – one which lasts longer than a few manicures
- a body brush – with natural bristles
- a hairdryer – especially if you have got mid-length to long hair
- a round or straightening hair brush – ditto

'until some bright spark brings back hair mascaras (such a great invention – whatever happened to them?), the best way to retouch your roots – something Sophie (39) wanted to find out – is to put Jolen on them with a toothbrush'

... and what you can probably do without

- eyelash curlers – you should not need them if you have got a good mascara.
- eyebrow brush (unless it comes on a wand in a brow groomer) – use your finger or an old toothbrush and a bit of hair gel, Vaseline or hairspray to push the hairs up.
- straightening irons – we know, we know, everyone says they are essentials. But poker-straight hair puts *years* on you and gives you a very hard look; softer straightness – achieved with a round or 'ironing' brush – is much, much more flattering. If you are going to use them though, get ceramic straightening irons; they are kinder on your hair.
- waxy crayons for removing make-up splodges: what is wrong with a cotton Q-tip and a bit of spit?

eyebrows

what's the big deal?

No one bothered with eyebrows for years – well, certainly not since the hippy Seventies when 'excess' hair growth was positively encouraged. But then suddenly no one can stop banging on about them and you can't open a magazine without getting tips on how to pluck and pull them to perfection. Why? Because – as anyone who has done it will tell you – shaping your brows, or even just tidying them up, has an *amazing* impact on your face. If the area beneath your brows is hair-free – and the arch is ever so slightly enhanced – it has the effect of 'opening' up your eyes and making the area look cleaner. And the overall impact on your face is de-ageing.

reshaping your brows If you have never bothered to pluck your brows we urge you to try it; you will be bowled over by the results. There are two ways to go about this. You can either get a professional to re-shape them for you (we would recommend this if your brows are quite bushy and unruly); or you can do the job yourself with a brow-shaping template (see our Best Beauty Accessory list on page 179). After that it is just a question of regularly tidying them up by plucking under and between them, but never above – unless you want to change their shape possibly forever.

tidying up your brows If this is all your brows need – do it! Just resist the temptation to overdo it. Plucking eyebrows can be like eating a bag of sherbet lemons: once you have started it can be tricky to stop.

hair

increasing the volume This is what most of us try to achieve when we blow-dry our hair – and how do we do it? Usually by flipping our heads upside-down and sticking the drier on full blast – which is fine, it works. But if you have got the right gadgets there are other easy ways to do it:

1. Rough-dry your hair with the hairdryer on high speed
2. Wind a few large Velcro rollers in the hair on the crown of your head, or if you have a fringe, put it in a roller
3. Blow-dry on a low to medium speed until your hair is bone dry (otherwise the effects will drop out quickly)
4. Leave the rollers in for about ten minutes when you have finished drying, then remove them and tease your hair into place

two simple shine-boosting tips To make your hair shine you need to get the cuticles on the strands to lie flat, so that light reflects more evenly off the surface and it looks shinier. To achieve this:

1. Do your last rinse after shampooing and conditioning with cool (or even better, cold) water – it can act like an astringent, shutting down the cuticles.
2. Hold your hairdryer so that it is pointing down the hair shaft from root to tip – another way to flatten the cuticle, and use it on a medium setting.

why the best place for nail scissors is in the bin

All good manicurists will tell you that the only way to keep your nails at a wearable length is to file them. Resist the urge to cut them – even if they get so long it takes ages to file them down again – as scissors split and traumatise nails. Even cuticle clippers should only be used in the rarest of circumstances – when part of your cuticle peels off and needs trimming. To stop the peeling off or splitting, keep your nails shaped in a practical 'squoval' (half square half oval) using the finest file you can lay your hands on, and rub a little nail oil into them and the cuticles whenever you remember.

the 9 best beauty accessories

the mission to find you the most effective and user-friendly beauty accessories on the market.

the criteria in order to be able to reveal which beauty gadgets are really worth buying, we used our own expertise, badgered all the professionals we know – hairstylists, make-up artists and beauty therapists – as well as asking our testers if there were any particular accessories they could not live without, to compile this road test. So what you have here are the staples you will find in every professional's kitbag.

Marian Newman's Everlasting Nail File £24.50

Marian Newman is a living legend, famous for her amazing nail creations for the catwalk. She is also a stickler for nail care, and designed this nail file – using toughened glass and Swarovski (yes, truly) crystals – to be abrasive enough to do the job, but fine too, so it does not traumatise your nails. The best thing about it? It lasts forever!

Elemis Body Brush £14.50

One body brush is much like another, isn't it? Er, well, no actually. If you are serious about body brushing (and you will be doing your skin and body a power of good if you do it regularly: the power of the humble body brush is such that you may find, after using it everyday for a month, you don't need expensive anti-cellulite creams) you need a decent brush. And in an ideal world it should have natural bristles and – this is *so key* – be designed so you can grip it properly: you have to be a contortionist to be able to do the job properly with a brush that has a handle!

Diamancel The Classic Big Buffer £39

No other foot file touches this in performance and yes, we know it is expensive, but we would not recommend it unless it was an investment that will last you forever. We all have hard skin on our feet – some of us worse than others – and foot files or buffers can transform them. Our tip is to file your feet very gently *after* a bath – not before one. Many people make this mistake and take too much skin off because it is hard and they don't feel it until they get in the bath. OUCH! This buffer has electro-plated diamond dust to work off dead skin and catch it so it doesn't go all over the place. Genius.

Tweezerman Slant Tweezer £16

You have probably read it before (and we wish we could be more imaginative on this) but these really are the king of tweezers. Why? Several reasons. Beautiful, well-shaped brows rely on precision plucking – something you can only achieve with sharp, shaped tweezers like these. Tweezers should be easy to grip (so not too short – those mini 'portable' ones are hopeless), allowing you to work quickly, grab a hair and pull it out cleanly, so you don't get left with awful red specks – the blood drawn by blunt tweezers and clumsy plucking. These tweezers deliver the goods, which is why you find them in every make-up artist's kitbag. They also come with a lifetime guarantee for free sharpening service.

Remington Bikini Trim & Shape

£19.99

This is the handy little gadget make-up artists pull out of their kitbags to deal with stray hairs when they are on some remote Polynesian beach helping with a bikini photo shoot for a magazine. If you don't want to go on holiday looking like an over-grown lawn – and you can't face a Brazilian (frankly the thought of them makes us feel faint – we are both far too English) – yet want a bikini-line effect to last longer than a razor job, this is the gadget to get. You use it on dry skin and there are five 'length' settings for the trimmer comb – or you can take the comb off for an even closer trim.. Best of all: it makes the process painless.

Mason Pearson Hairbrush

£41.50 for the handy version

The classic hairbrush – you can't beat Mason Pearson brushes – and you will see the mini ones in all the best hairstylist's back pockets. It has straight, natural pure boar bristles mixed with pure nylon. It comes in four sizes – pocket, handy, medium and large.

Denman Ceramic Straightening Brush

£8

Kate claims that this hair ironing brush changed her life. It makes lighter work of straightening thick and wavy hair than a circular brush and achieves a much more flattering effect than straightening irons because it straightens your hair softly – it doesn't make it poker straight which adds years to your face and pulls down your features. This brush has aluminium plates insulated by a thermo ceramic coating, which protects hair from heat damage, and a vent within the bristles makes warm air circulate more freely, drying your hair faster.

Andrew Collinge Professional 1800W

£24.99

A famous hairdresser's name on the side of a dryer doesn't make a scrap of difference to its performance: all you need is a dryer that is light to hold and powerful. Which is exactly what this is. It has three heat settings – including a cool shot (great for flattening cuticles and boosting shine) – and two speed settings.

Denman Thermo Magic Rollers

£4.50 per pack

No, rollers did not go out with the Ark: they are key if you want to give your hair extra volume or bounce. There is a big difference between modern rollers and the ones your mother used: rollers don't need pins or grips to hold them in anymore – not if you get a good set anyway – and these self-fixing ones don't just stay in your hair by themselves, they self-heat too. We think they are the best you can buy.

BEAUTY LEXIS: making real sense of beauty speak

How many of these beauty catchphrases and ingredients can you honestly say you understand the meaning of: anti-ageing, liposomes, alpha hydroxy acids (AHAs), exfoliation, animal friendly. Two? Three? All of them?

Our guess is that you have probably heard of them all at some point but are only familiar with a couple. But then it wouldn't surprise us to hear that you haven't got a clue what any of them really mean.

Beauty has its own unique language based on buzzwords which evolve with new ingredients, formulas and techniques, and which are often manipulated to mean different things for different purposes. This is why most of us only have the vaguest idea of what they mean or how they benefit us (or not, as the case may be). Several of our testers said they wished that products could explain what they did – and what they contained – in plain English, rather than scientific jargon and psychobabble.

The beauty houses don't necessarily mislead us on purpose, but they do single out and use words such as 'liposome' on packaging to make products sound swankier and more effective. Which may well be the case: some creams containing liposomes (or other popular anti-ageing ingredients like antioxidants and retin-A) might work better than those that don't. But this isn't necessarily a result of these ingredients alone.

The ingredient list on packaging isn't much help; you could be forgiven for thinking you need a degree in biochemistry to understand it what it means: how are you supposed to know what hyaluronic acid, AHAs, compounds and botanical complexes do? A few of our testers pointed this out, with Sue (40) asking, 'Do they blind us with science on purpose because they think we will take it as read that the ingredients are good for us and therefore buy their products?'

You rarely get a full or totally impartial explanation of what each ingredient does that goes into a beauty product (and that ultimately goes on *you*) – or for that matter, of the claims made by beauty products. Which is why this bit of the book is so key. We believe that unless you understand the basics of beauty speak you can't make informed decisions about products and whether you need – or want – them.

So even if you reckon you could sit an exam on all the latest buzzwords don't skip this bit. The information we give you here is, like the rest of the information in the book, the most honest and impartial you are likely to get.

It will give you a better understanding of the language on which the whole beauty business is based. Be prepared for a few surprises – some of the following may be eye-opening ...

algae – is seaweed, and it is often applied to beauty products (especially genuine 'spa' ones) because it is full of nutrients that are said to be good for your skin and body.

alpha hydroxy acids (AHAs) – are a group of acids extracted from foods such as fruit, milk and wine and are used as active 'anti-ageing' ingredients in body lotions, face creams, serums, masks and cleansers. They have two roles: they make skin smooth and increase cell turnover. So if you have ever wondered why the Romans splashed red wine on their faces – or why Cleopatra bathed in asses' milk – this is the answer. This is also why you find ingredients such as papaya and grapefruit in cleansers: they make products smell nice and fresh, yes, but they also have a physiological effect on your skin.

animal friendly – a big and complex minefield! And one which many of the people who did our survey asked us to explain. Others said they didn't want to test products which were not animal friendly or had been tested on animals. Some of you (rightly) said that labelling should be clearer as to whether or not products had been tested on animals. Animal testing is too big a topic for us to explain fully here. But what we can say in this space is that *all ingredients – natural or not – have been tested on animals at some point in time,* and often not by the company that has manufactured the product but by a separate laboratory. Which should give you plenty of food for thought.

anti-ageing – there are so many interpretations of this little term that it isn't surprising many people are baffled by or have unrealistic expectations of the benefits of anti-ageing products. Anti-ageing, time-fighting, de-ageing – they all mean the same thing: that a product either aims to delay premature ageing (and this is *preventable* ageing caused by factors such as cigarettes, stress and UV light, not uncontrollable influences like your genes) by protecting skin with a UV filter, or, by using an active anti-ageing ingredient (a 'cosmeceutical' – a cross between a cosmetic and a pharmaceutical), has a physiological impact on your skin, making age signs such as fine lines look less visible. Anti-ageing does not mean that a product will completely reverse all signs of time on your face.

antioxidant – describes what an ingredient *does.* In beauty products antioxidants such as vitamins A, C and E and grape seed extract (there are thousands of ingredients with antioxidant properties) are said to neutralise free radicals, the reactive molecules that wrinkle your skin. But the jury is still out on how much topically applied antioxidants are required to be effective.

aromatherapy oils – also known as essential oils, these are extracted from plants and put into beauty products as they have therapeutic properties on mind and body.

beta hydroxy acid (BHAs) – such as salicylic acid are found in natural sources like willow bark and have similar effects as AHAs but work on a deeper level.

botanicals – are plants and plant extracts which are added to beauty products for their beneficial qualities. It is worth bearing in mind that although a botanical such as white lily extract might sound better for you than a chemical such as L-ascorbic or hyaluronic acid, this isn't necessarily the case.

ceramides – these are often included in anti-ageing creams because they are said to help to strengthen your skin's natural barrier, thus helping keep in essential moisture.

collagen & elastin – often described as the skin's 'scaffolding' or 'mattressing', they are a network of cross-linked fibres beneath the skin which support it and make it supple and pingy. The fibres diminish with age, which is why many anti-ageing creams contain synthetic collagen or ingredients such as vitamin C which are said to encourage collagen production.

emollients – these are skin-softeners and most creams and cosmetics (especially the thicker ones) contain them. There are lots of different types with long and/or hi-tech names such as PEG-60 hydrogenated castor oil and stearic acid. It's usually best for people with very oily skin to avoid emollient creams because the ingredient is similar to natural oil or sebum and thus might add to the problem.

enzymes – are extracted from fruit such as papaya (papain, an enzyme found in at least two of the body exfoliators we tested, is extracted from unripe papayas) and exfoliate the skin like AHAs, but tend to be more mild.

free radicals – are the reactive molecules that age your skin and you. Free radicals are generated by factors such as the sun's ultraviolet (UV) rays, cigarette smoke and even stress. Their effects – a gradual degeneration of the body – happen over a long period of time, which is why it is so hard to measure the reversal effect of antioxidant ingredients in beauty products on the skin.

glycerine – is a useful humectant which, when added to moisturiser, can help bind moisture into the tissues.

grape & grape seed extract – are very potent antioxidants, which is why they are some of the sexiest beauty ingredients of the moment.

human growth factor (HGF) – these are from a family of hormones produced by the body to control cell growth, and when applied to state-of-the-art anti-ageing creams they may promote repair.

hyaluronic acid – a polysaccharide found naturally in the body's connective tissues and used in skin creams because it is a potent moisturiser.

hypo-allergenic – another confusing term and open to various interpretations. It usually means that a product has been screened for ingredients that commonly cause irritancy; so it may or may not exclude a property that annoys your skin.

lanolin – is one of the best moisturisers a cream can contain, but has been burdened for years (unfairly, we think) with a reputation for causing sensitivity.

light reflection – products (mostly cosmetics but moisturisers and most skin primers too) which are light-reflective contain tiny optical diffusers, particles which deflect light away from the skin in a way that flatters it and plays down blemishes and fine lines. Iridescent products can also have this effect.

liposomes – are often used to market beauty products in a way that suggests they are miracle anti-ageing ingredients, when in fact it is what is *inside them* that counts more than liposomes themselves. Liposomes are tiny inert 'bubbles' – nothing more complex that that – which scientists fill with active anti-ageing ingredients in the hope that they will carry these deeper into your skin. So liposomes are a form of transport – an ingredient bus if you like – and companies have developed their own varieties ('micelles' and 'hydrobeads'). It is debatable whether or not they make anti-ageing products more effective.

mineral oil & petrolatum – are often included in super-hydrating balms and creams. They are a cheap substitute for natural oils, but while some beauty scientists believe that they block pores because they are not absorbed and sit like a film on your skin, most say they are the safest, most non-irritating agents used in beauty.

natural – a well-used word in beauty today with *huge* marketing clout but quite a hazy definition too because the term can imply different things and may be used even if a product has only one natural ingredient in it – or *none at all*. Amazing, but true. Products with botanical extracts in them are often called 'natural', but very few – if any – are all-natural. How could they be? If a product contained no preservatives it would go off and no one wants to put mouldy cream on their face. 'Natural' ingredients such as botanical extracts are not always better than chemicals; they are not automatically organic and should not cost any more money than regular products.

non-comedogenic – a very long word for a product specially developed not to block pores and cause spots or make acne worse.

olive oil – has antioxidant qualities and is very moisturising, which is why it is increasingly found in face creams.

organic – was another misused word until April 2002 when the Soil Association introduced its own Health & Beauty Standards guidelines to ensure that organic ranges are truly organic. The guidelines ban certain ingredients such as the foaming agents sodium lauryl sulphate and sodium laureth sulphate, allow no genetically modified ingredients or any testing on animals. See the box on page 187 for ranges that have been awarded the Organic Standard label.

retin-A – see vitamin A.

sun protection factor (SPF) – this denotes the amount of protection a sunscreen, cosmetic or beauty product gives you. The higher the number the higher the protection.

tea (green, black & white) – contains polyphenols which are powerful antioxidants with anti-inflammatory benefits.

vitamin A – the technical name for vitamin A is retinol, and it hit the headlines as a magic ingredient for prescription anti-ageing products back in 1987. The main benefit it has is on your skin's texture – it makes it much smoother, and can visibly soften lines and deeper wrinkles. It is worth bearing in mind though that although they are derivatives of vitamin A – and sound similar – retin-A, retinyl palmitate and Renova are not the same ingredients as retinol.

vitamin C – isn't just a cure for a cold! It can also promote formation of collagen – the stuff that makes your skin springy – when applied topically, and it has antioxidant properties. This is why it is added – in different forms (such as L-ascorbic acid and magnesium ascorbyl phosphate) – to anti-ageing treatments.

vitamin E – a well-known antioxidant. Also called alpha tocopherol, it protects cells from free radical damage and is used in about eight different forms (including tocotrienols) in – usually – time-fighting beauty products.

organic beauty ranges

These ranges have been awarded the Soil Association's Organic Standard label. Refer to the Beauty Store on page 188 for contact details:

Aromatherapy oils

Absolute Aromas
Aladdin Aromas
Baldwins
The Organic Herb Trading Co

Bath, massage and essential oils

Health Quest Ltd
Mill House Farm Molyneux Medicinal & Aromatic Plant Farm
New Seasons
NHR Organics
Paul Richards Herbal Supplies
Spiezia Organics

Beauty, health and baby care products

Green People
Neal's Yard Remedies
Spiezia Organics

touchy ingredients

In the responses we got to our questionnaires lots of people said they thought some ingredients sounded 'toxic' and 'too chemical' – and asked whether any should be avoided. There is controversy over some ingredients – we won't deny it – but only *you* can decide whether it bothers you enough to avoid using the products that contain these ingredients altogether.

Here are some of the 'hottest' ingredients:

DEA (diethanolamine) – a study done in America in 1999 found an association between cancer and the application of DEA-related ingredients in tests. Although it is found in many different products – from bubble bath and shampoo, to hair dye, conditioner and dishwasher liquid – it is only used in tiny amounts, and has not been declared an official health hazard by cosmetic monitoring bodies.

formaldehyde – also known as toluene, it is a toughening property in nail care products, but it can also make nails dry, which is why some people like to avoid nail polishes that contain it. As toluene it has a more chequered history. Claims have been made in America that it is hazardous to health, but Samantha Sweet, director of Creative Nails says tests have proved that 'the amount of toluene present in a "busy salon" is almost 200 times below the limits deemed safe'.

lanolin – is a fantastic emollient in creams but has had a reputation for years for causing sensitivity, even though recorded cases of this are very low.

oxygen – is applied to some skin care products via hydrogen peroxide which releases an oxygen molecule when it comes into contact with your skin; this is thought to delay ageing because oxygen in your skin depletes with age. However, exposure to oxygen also *ages* your skin by triggering free radicals, which is why oxygen creams have always been quite a puzzling development.

SD alcohol – can cause sensitivity. Our advice is to use quantity as your guide; products usually contain more of it when it is at the top of the ingredient list.

sodium lauryl sulphate (SLS) & sodium laureth sulphate (SLES) – although SLS has been known to irritate skin, the claim that SLS and SLES could cause cataracts was actually an unsubstantiated rumour that started in America.

talc – a lot of people don't use face powder because of talc's apparent health implications. However, more research needs to be done to prove whether or not it does cause health problems.

BEAUTY STORE: where to find everything

These are the contact details for all the products and brands mentioned in *Beauty Scoop*. Most companies offer a mail order service – either over the phone or on their websites (not all websites offer a purchasing service) – some will direct you to your nearest stockist of their products and others are able to offer you advice on using their products.

A

absolute aromas: ☎01420 540400 / www.absolute-aromas.com
aladdin aromas: ☎01434 382820 / www.aladdinaromas.co.uk
almay: ☎0800 085 2716 / www.almay.com
amanda lacey: ☎020 7370 4410 / www.amandalacy.com
amirose: ☎020 8554 3335 / www.amirose.com
andrew collinge: ☎0151 709 5942 / www.andrewcollinge.com
aromatherapy associates: ☎020 8569 7030 / www.aromatherapyassociates.com
astor: available at Boots and Superdrug nationwide
aussie: ☎0191 297 5000 / www.aussie.com
australian bodycare: ☎01892 750333 / www.australianbodycare.co.uk
aveda: ☎01730 232380 / www.aveda.com
avèue: ☎0845 1170116
avon: ☎0845 601 3371 / www.avon.uk.com

B

b kamins: ☎020 7299 4999 / www.b.kamins.com
babyliss: ☎0870 5133191 / www.babyliss.com
badger: ☎01543 480100 / www.graftons.co.uk
baldwins: ☎020 7703 5550 / www.baldwins.co.uk
barbara daly: ☎0800 505535 / available from Tesco
barielle: ☎020 7636 0234 / www.barielleinternational.com
becca: ☎020 7299 4999 & 0870 169 9999 / www.beccacosmetics.com
benefit: ☎09011 130001 / www.benefitcosmetics.com
big sexy hair: ☎020 8381 7793 / www.sexyhairconcepts
bio-col marine: ☎0845 0754544 / www.biocol.co.uk
bioré: available from chemists nationwide / www.biore.com
black like me: ☎020 8988 8550 / www.blacklikeme.co.za
bliss: ☎020 7584 3888 / www.blissworld.com
blistex: available from supermarkets and chemists nationwide / www.blistex.com
bobbi brown: ☎01730 232566 / www.bobbibrowncosmetics.com
body shop: ☎020 7208 7966 / www.thebodyshop.com
boots: ☎0845 0708090 / www.boots-plc.com & www.wellbeing.com
borghese: ☎01273 408800 / www.borghese.com
bourjois: ☎0800 269 8386 / www.bourjois.com

C

caudalie: ☎020 7304 7038 / www.caudalie.com
cellex c: ☎08457 402214 / www.cellex-cuk.com
chanel: ☎020 7493 3836 / www.chanel.com
chantecaille: ☎020 7629 9161 & 020 7636 4686
charles worthington: ☎020 7636 4686 / www.cwlondon.com
christian breton: ☎01322 290101 / www.christian-breton.com
christian dior: ☎01932 233902 / www.dior.com
circaroma: ☎020 7249 9392 / www.circaroma.com
citre shine: available from Boots nationwide / www.citreshine.com
clarins: ☎0800 036 3558 / www.clarins.com
clinique: ☎01730 232566 / www.clinique.com
collection 2000: ☎0870 755 1055
cosmetics a la carte: ☎020 7622 2318 / www.cosmeticsalacarte.com
crabtree & evelyn: ☎020 7603 1611 / www.crabtree-evelyn.com
creative nail design: ☎0113 274 8486 / www.creativenail.com
crème de la mer: ☎01730 232 566/ www.gloss.com

D

daniel galvin: ☎020 7486 9661 / www.daniel-galvin.co.uk
darphin: ☎020 8847 1877 / www.darphin.fr
ddf (doctor's dermalogic formula): ☎020 7235 5000 / www.ddfskin.com
decleor: ☎020 7402 9474 / www.decleor.com
denman: ☎0800 262509 / www.denmanbrush.com

dermablend: 0870 8377377 / www.dermablend.com
dermalogica: 0800591 818 / www.dermalogica.com
diamancel: 0808 100 4151 / www.diamancel.com
diprobase: available from chemists nationwide

E

e'spa: 01252 42800 / www.espaonline.com
eau thermale avene: 0845 117 0116
elemis: 020 8954 8033 / www.elemis.com
elizabeth arden: 020 7574 2700 / www.elizabetharden.com
ella baché: 01753 880537 / www.ellabache.citysearch.com
epure: 020 7620 1771
estée lauder: 01730 232566 / www.esteelauder.com
eve lom: 020 8661 7991 / 0870 169 9999 / www.evelom.com
eyeko: 020 7734 9090 / www.eyebeautyusa.com

F

farmacia: 020 7404 8808 / www.farmacia.co.uk
fresh: 08708 377377 / www.fresh.com

G

gatineau: 0800 731 5805 / www.thebeautyroom.com
gillette: 00800 44553883 / www.gillette.com
givenchy: 020 7730 1234/ www.givenchy.com
green people: 01444 401444 / www.greenpeople.co.uk
guerlain: 01932 233874 / www.guerlain.com

H

hair solutions: available from Boots nationwide
hard candy: 08450 708090 / www.hardcandy.com
hardys: 01223 441821
health quest ltd: 020 8206 2066 / www.healthquest.co
helena rubinstein: 020 8762 4040 / www.helenarubinstein.com

I

i coloniali: 020 7297 5000 / www.icoloniali.com
i.d bareminerals: 0870 850 6655 / www.bareescentuals.com
iman: 01280 707 499 / www.i-iman.com

J

jessica: 020 8381 7793 / www.jessicacosmetics.com
john frieda: 020 7245 0033 / www.johnfrieda.com
jolen: available from chemists nationwide
jurlique: 020 8841 6644 / www.jurlique.com.au

K

kerastase: 0800 316 4400/ www.kerastase.com
keromask: 01252 533349
kiehl's: 020 7240 2411 / www.kiehls.com
know how: 020 7935 0982 / www.knowhowhair.com

L

l'oréal: 0845 399 1959 / www.lorealparis.com
la prairie: 020 8398 5300 / www.laprairie.com
lamberts: 01892 552117 / www.naturesbestonline.com
lancaster: 0800 376 0688 / www.lancaster-beauty.com
lancome: 020 8762 4040 / www.lancome.com
laura mercier: 0870 169 9999 / www.lauramercier.com
leirac: 020 7620 1771
liz earle: 01983 813913 / www.lizearle.net
lush: 01202 668 545 / www.lush.com

M

mac cosmetics: 020 7534 9222 / www.maccosmetics.com
makeup for ever: 020 7529 5690 / www.makeupforever.com
malki: 020 8203 6643 / www.deadseabath.co.uk
marian newman: 07740 873378
marks & spencer: 0845 3021234 / www.marksandspencer.com
mary cohr: 0808 100 3102
mason pearson: 020 7491 2613 / www.masonpearson.com
matis: 01322 290101 / www.matis-uk.com
max factor: 0800 169 1302 / www.maxfactor.com
mayaltha: 01280 70749 / www.mayaltha.com
maybelline: 0845 399 0304 / www.maybelline.com
md formulations: 01268 724411
michaeljohn: 020 7491 4401 /available from Boots nationwide
mill house farm molyneux medicinal & aromatic plant farm: 0151 526 0139 /www.m www.phytobotanica.com
molton brown: 020 7499 6474 / www.moltonbrown.com

N

nads: 0870 7280683 / www.nads.co.uk
nails inc: 020 7499 8333 / www.nailsinc.com
nailtiques: 01543 480 100 / www.nailtiques.com
neal's yard remedies: 020 7627 1949 / www.nealsyardremedies.com
neutrogena: 01628 822 2222 / www.neutrogena.com
new seasons: 01235 821110 / www.newseasons.co.uk
nexxus: 01752 222 177 / www.nexxus.com
nhr organics: 08453 108066 / www.nhrorganicoils.com

nicky clarke hairomatherapy: 0845 601 4634 / www.nickyclarke.co.uk
nivea: 0800 616977 / www.nivea.com
no7: 08450 708090 / www.boots-plc.com / www.wellbeing.com
norgrow: 01945 410810 / www.norgrow.com

O

oenobiol: 0870 837 7377 / www.oenobiol.fr
origins: 0800 731 4039 / www.origins.com
olay: 0800 917 7197 / www.olay.com
omega ingredients: 01728 726 626 / www.omegaingredients.co
opi: 01923 240010 / www.opi.com
optrex: 0115 968 8664/ www.optrexeyes.com
organic pharmacy: 020 7351 2232 / theorganicpharmacy.com
origins: 0800 731 4039 / www.origins.com
over the top: 0871 220 4141 / www.hqhair.com

P

pantene: 0800 0283378 / www.pantene.com
paul mitchell: 01296 390 590 / www.paulmitchell.com
paul richards herbal supplies: 01544 327 360
philosophy: 0845 070 9080 / www.philosophy.com
phytomer: 0808 100 2204 / www.phytomer.com
pixi: 020 7287 7211 / www.pixibeauty.com
pout: 020 7379 0379 / www.pout.co.uk
ponds: 020 8439 6000 / www.ponds.com
prescriptives: 01730 232 566 / www.gloss.com/px
papa: 01932 254854
pure hair: 01277 263366 / www.arteceurope.com

Q

qvc the shopping channel: 0800 50 40 30 / www.qvcuk.com

R

re vive: 0870 169 9999
redken: 0800 44 880 / www.redken.com
reimann: 01634 226203 / www.p20.co.uk
remington: 0800 212 438 / www.remingtonbikini.co.uk
ren: 020 7935 2323 / www.ren.ltd.uk
revlon: 0800 085 2716 / www.revlon.com
rimmel: 020 8971 1300 / www.rimmellondon.com
rmk: 020 7235 5000 / www.rmkrmk.com
roc: 0845 6004477 / www.roc.com
rose & co apothecary: 01535 646830 / www.rose-apothecary.co.uk
ruby & millie: 08450 450 708090 / www.boots.com

S

sally hansen: 01252 533349 / www.sallyhansen.com
sex symbol: 020 8381 7793
shiseido: 020 7836 5588 / www.shiseido.co.uk
shu uemura: 020 7379 6627 / www.shu-uemura.co.jp
sisley: 020 7491 2722 / www.sisley-cosmetics.com
sixtus: 020 8979 7261
skin wisdom: 0800 505535 / www.tesco.com
spiezia organics: 01326 231 600 / www.spieziaorganics.com
st tropez: 0115 983 6363 / www.sttropez.co.uk
stila: 01730 232566 / www.stilacosmetics.com
superdrug: 0800 0961055 / www.superdrug.com
supernail of LA: 020 8752 1924 / www.supernail.co.uk

T

talika: 0870 169 9999 / www.talika.com
thalgo: 0800 146041 / www.thalgo.co.uk
the body shop: 01903 731500 / www.thebodyshop.com
the lift: 01926 438 540
the organic herb trading co: 01823 401 205 / www.organicherbtrading.com
the soil association: 0117 929 0661 / www.soilassociation.org
tigi: 020 8388 1300 / wwwtigihaircare.com
trevor sorbie: 01372 375235 / www.trevorsorbie.com
tweezerman: 0207 252 7046 / www.tweezerman.com

U

ultima ii: 0800 085 2716 / www.revlon.co.uk
umberto giannini: 01384 444771 / www.umbertogiannini.com

V

vaseline: 0800 591 720 / www.vaseline.com
veet: 0845 769 7079 / www.veet.inquiries.co.uk
vichy: 0800 169 6193 / www.vichy.com
virgin vie: 0845 300 8022 / www.virgin.com/cosmetics

W

wu: 0870 241 4902 / www.mankindonline.co.uk

Y

yves saint laurent: 01444 255700 / www.ysl.com

NB: all prices and contact details are correct at the time of publication.

THE TOP 10 BEAUTY COMMANDMENTS: how to turn yourself into a discerning beauty shopper!

THOU SHALT NOT

1. believe that expensive products are automatically better than inexpensive ones: sometimes they are, but women who spend lots of money on cosmetics do not necessarily have better skin, hair or bodies than those who don't.
2. believe that 'natural' beauty products are better than regular beauty products.
3. believe that an anti-ageing product can completely erase your wrinkles.
4. believe that an anti-cellulite cream can completely remove cellulite by tackling it from the outside in.
5. believe *everything* a sales assistant tells you.
6. look at pictures of teenage models (photographed in manipulated light) and pampered celebrities (who have hairstylists, dieticians, make-up artists and clothes stylists on hand 24/7) and believe that is how your skin, hair or body should – or *will* – look after you have bought the product they are endorsing or advertising. It will not.
7. be seduced by every new promotion, product or concept that the beauty industry decides to throw at you; instead buy the products *you* need and want.
8. sit in the sun unprotected: you won't just end up with skin like an old leather boot, but greatly raise your risk of getting skin cancer too, especially if you are pale-skinned.
9. smoke. Ditto above (until you stop you don't realise how much of an impact smoking has on your looks) together with the obvious health reasons.
10. shop for beauty products without the confidence to know what you do or don't need. Our aim is to turn you into an informed shopper, because if you are not, it can cost you dearly, believe us. NB: *Beauty Scoop* is specially made to fit in your handbag!

ACKNOWLEDGEMENTS

The following 257 friends, friends of friends, acquaintances, work colleagues and family spent much of last year testing over 2,000 beauty products for us and filling in our lengthy questionnaires to tell us what they thought of the products they had tried. It is a cliché, but there is no other way to say it: without their cooperation and goodwill this book really *really* could not have been written. So a big thank you to:

Alice Guillemet, Alice Peterson, Alice Valdes-Scott, Alicky Gravell, Allie Mayhew, Amanda Ingleby, Amanda Wiltshire, Andrea Simmonds, Angela Cary, Angela Knowlton, Angela Vose, Angie Douglas, Anna Power, Anna Raymond, Anna Speer, Annabel Holland, Annabelle Dodd, Annalise Malloy, Anne Lawrence, Anne Smith, Anneka Meade, Anneka Rouch, Annette Jacobs, Annie Cawley, Annie Morgan, Annya Parson, Bridget Reading, Bronwyn Richards, Candice Juniper, Candice Warner, Carina Cowan, Caroline Benny, Caroline Boyle, Caroline Browne, Caroline Dewar, Caroline Mann, Caroline Sanders, Caroline Wilson, Catherine Airlie, Catherine Davies, Cathy Andrews, Cathy Kusmirek, Cathy Wilson, Ceire Clark, Chris Acland, Christina Hicks, Christina Howard, Christine Matheson, Cindy Parkes, Claire Hutton, Claire Sands, Clare Clark, Clare Grogan, Dawn Mills, Dawn McArthur, Dean Fawley, Debbie Gorse, Debbie Hislop, Deborah Idiens, Dede Crossley, Dee Brand, Denise Bates, Dierdre Moran, Dierdre Wade, Doreen Parr, Eliza Bennett, Elizabeth Coles, Emillie Ruston, Emily Fisher, Emma Douglas, Emma Heyman, Emma Hughes, Emma Samonians, Emma Wyndham Blake, Eve Threlkeld, Faye Ashton, Fi Hunter-Inglis, Fi Kent, Frances Keegan, Genevieve Dolittle, Georgiana Bray, Georgie Brooke, Gill Howe, Hannah McMichael, Hannah Riddle, Harriet Camperner, Heather Conlon, Heather Peerman, Helen Morton, Helena Catlin, Helena Keene, Heloise Spence, Helsie Noel, Hilary North, Hilary Wayland, Iona Jolls, Isabel Albiston, Imogen Marks, Isabel Sheehy, Jackie Hyde, Jackie Noel, Jacqueline Fielding, Jane Auer, Jane Hollyman, Jane Moore, Jane Roberts, Jane Rose, Janey Davis, Janey Warburton, Jennifer Crisp, Jennifer Warner, Jenny House, Jill Moores, Jo Andrews, Jo Eke, Jo Lloyd, Joan Linehan, Joanna Burns, Josie Carter, Josie Orbach, Joy Smith, Julia Dixon, Julia Rhodes, Julianna Thompson, Julie Surman, Juliet Caulfield, Juliet Keene, June Derby, June Walker, Karen Silver, Karen Mearn-Bray, Kari Lerner, Kate Cazenove, Kate Raby-Smith, Kate Ward, Katie Marshall, Katie de'Ath, Kerry Moore, Kirsty Milner, Laura Mason, Laura Pickering, Lauren Taylor, Leah McCreeth, Libby Harris, Lily Stevens, Linda Carpenter, Linda Raine, Lindsay Hamilton, Lisa Greenwood, Lisa Harold, Lisa John, Lisa Williams, Liz Hughes, Liza Duffy, Lizzie Raban, Lorna Duffy, Lottie Clayburn, Lottie Riza, Lou Pearce, Lou Walmsley, Louise Carpenter, Louise Murphy, Louise Pentland-Murray, Loulie Hollis, Lucinda de Mauley, Lucy Barkman, Lucy Doggrel, Lucy Peck, Lucy Shapland, Luke Greenwood, Magda Kowalik-Malcolm, Magda Maron, Margaret Doherty, Margaret Hill, Margaret Hope, Maria Brannigan, Maria Mckay, Marina Hansen, Mary-Ann Seymour, Maureen Aston, Maxine Tallon, Mel Paige, Melanie Cantor, Melissa Bryden, Michelle White, Milly Herbert, Misba Alvi, Molly Wilks, Myra Brown, Nancy Wickens, Natalie Roberts, Nicky Teeks, Nicola Blacoe, Nina Murray, Nourdjan Parmenter, Olivia Galvin, Pamela Malcolm, Paula Denning, Paula Downes, Pauline Wilkes, Philippa Wiggin, Philly Coates, Philly Hamner, Polly Ward, Rosemary Cairns, Ruth Groves, Saba Syed, Sal Brooks, Sally Barber, Sally Talbot, Sam Lane, Sam Sheaff, Sam Warleigh, Sammy Hayden, Sammy Keene, Sandra Harrison, Sandra Smith, Sara Kaye-Johnson, Sarah Cameron, Sarah Harris, Sarah Hart, Sarah Hurt, Sarah Maynard, Sarah Ruff, Sarah Savitt, Sarah Woods, Sarah-Jane Hall, Sasha Meera, Shauna Lowry, Shirley Hall, Simon Greenwood, Sophie Brown, Sophie Janes, Sophie Northam, Sue Meade, Sue Whitley, Susie Peacock, Suzanne Kurtz, Tamsin Moore, Tania Brown, Tara Johnson, Tessa Little, Tina Edgson, Toni Lazerus, Trudie Dyer, Trudy Meyer, Valencia Haynes, Vicki McIvor, Vickie Hindmarch, Vicky Henderson, Victoria Rush, Victoria Tydeman, Victoria Wayland-Smith and Zoe Pace.

We also want to say a special thank you to Denise Bates, Illustrated Publishing Director at Collins, for her supreme patience and hand-holding; to Magda Kowalik-Malcolm, who helped co-ordinate the massive beauty road test and spent weeks packing up and sending out parcels full of products for us; to the beauty press offices who supplied us with products; and most of all to those closest to us: Ben and Molly, Rob, Honor, baby Florence (who arrived in the middle of the road test) and Biff – all of whom had to live for months on end in homes that were a cross between the chemist and the post office. And all in the name of BEAUTY! Thank you.